I0072932

Approaches to Health of Individuals Living in Different Cultures in Turkey

Fatma Eti Aslan (ed.)

Approaches to Health of Individuals Living in Different Cultures in Turkey

PETER LANG

**Bibliographic Information published by the
Deutsche Nationalbibliothek**
The Deutsche Nationalbibliothek lists this publication in the Deutsche
Nationalbibliografie; detailed bibliographic data is available online at
http://dnb.d-nb.de.

Library of Congress Cataloging-in-Publication Data
A CIP catalog record for this book has been applied for at the
Library of Congress.

The views expressed in this book are purely that of the author herself
and may not in any circumstances be regarded as stating an official
position of Bahçeşehir University.

ISBN 978-3-631-79217-9 (Print)
E-ISBN 978-3-631-80259-5 (E-PDF)
E-ISBN 978-3-631-80260-1 (EPUB)
E-ISBN 978-3-631-80261-8 (MOBI)
DOI 10.3726/b16161

© Peter Lang GmbH
Internationaler Verlag der Wissenschaften
Berlin 2019
All rights reserved.

Peter Lang – Berlin · Bern · Bruxelles · New York · Oxford · Warszawa · Wien

All parts of this publication are protected by copyright. Any
utilisation outside the strict limits of the copyright law, without
the permission of the publisher, is forbidden and liable to
prosecution. This applies in particular to reproductions,
translations, microfilming, and storage and processing in
electronic retrieval systems.

This publication has been peer reviewed.

www.peterlang.com

Foreword

It is the way of life of cultures that affect the perception of individuals' health. It is also determined by the cultural practices of health societies affected by biological and environmental factors. Each individual can define to be healthy differently based on their own values and beliefs. The perception of health is influenced by society, current social status and familial features. The concept of disease as well as health is influenced by these processes and can change all of the life balances of individuals. Cultural variables can be mobilizing factors in the health-disease relationship. Today, health-related cultural features are under the influence of a medical understanding that is almost all over the world. Health- and disease-related processes, perception of medical terms and the tendency to evaluate in this framework are increasing. Modern medicine consumes people's will to live their own realities and solve their problems. However, the concept of health should be taken away from a number of thought patterns and considered as a dynamic phenomenon in life. Therefore, in order to adopt the art of healthy living, health needs to be assessed with a comprehensive understanding of culture. It is important to know the cultural characteristics of the community to allow individuals and societies to participate by accepting this service in order to provide them with the desired level of health care. The conditions that are culturally important are generally overlooked in the presentation of health services, providing a proper cultural health care, understanding the dimensions of culture, leading to a holistic approach more than bio physicality, increasing knowledge, changing approaches and improving clinical skills.

This book is written by people who have experienced it in order to guide their health service servers. I believe that all readers will bring a scientific view of the pain and thank everyone who contributed to it.

Prof. Dr. Fatma Eti Aslan and Dr. Fadime Çınar

Contents

1 Culture and Health Relationship

1.1 Introduction

In response to the creations of nature, all kinds of values, beliefs, attitudes and behaviors, and customs are defined as "culture", which can be found, learned, shared and transferred between generations[1]. Culture is a share of values, beliefs, attitudes and behaviors that are learned, taught and transmitted from generation to generations[2]. It serves as an important tool in shaping and interpreting the environment in order to preserve human health, to ensure its welfare and to maintain its existence by transferring these shares, which will ensure the continuity of life.

We live in a global world where people's interactions from different cultures are increasing every day. Globalization; it brings economic, social, political and cultural ties between the various regions of the world. In addition, there are many changes in the economic, political, social, social and health fields[3,4,5]. It is important to be aware of the cultural differences and their effects among people in such a world. In the last century, in almost all regions of the world, together with globalization, wars, ethnic conflicts, environmental crises, suppressing regimes, economic collapse, as well as immigrant asylum seekers in many people, country or other countries or forced immigration. In this case, the multicultural population structures formed by individuals, families and groups from different cultures and

1 Şahin, N. H., Bayram, G. O., & Avcı, D. (2009). Culture-sensitive approach: transcultural nursing. *Koç University Journal of Education and Research in Nursing (NERJ)*, 6 (1), 2–7.
2 Bolsoy, N., & Sevil, Ü. (2006). Health-disease and culture interaction. *Journal of Ataturk University School of Nursing*, 9(3), 78–87.
3 Aksoy, Z. (2013). *Role of Cultural Intelligence in Multicultural Environments.* Unpublished PhD Thesis, Ege University Institute of Social Sciences, Public Relations and Publicity, İzmir.
4 Erdem, N., & Karaca Sivrikaya, S. (2015). Intercultural approach in the care of internal disease patients. Turkey Clinics. *Journal of Public Health Nursing-Special Topics*, 1(3), 14–21.
5 Held, D. (2010). *Globalization, Sociology: Initial Readings.* (A. Giddens, Ed.) (2nd ed.). İstanbul: Say Publications.

subcultures are emerging in the world[6,7]. The situation now focuses on the world's health policy approaches in recent years, primarily to prevent inequality and discrimination in ethnic traits and health[8]. Complex, similar and diverse cultural insights are common in multicultural societies based on cultural diversity. These are cultural insights; it is shaped by many factors such as age, gender, race, ethnic characteristics, socio-economic class, religious identity, religious rituals, education, etc. In other words, each individual perceives the world from its own culture window.

Due to the global world and the conditions it brings with it, it is necessary for the different cultural groups to live together or to establish intercultural interactions with health professionals for a number of reasons. The health team has highly increased the importance of raising health professionals who are well-known for their culture and who are equipped with cultural knowledge and skills to meet the cultural needs of societies. For this reason, it is necessary to recognize, be sensitive to and respect the cultural differences of individuals within the community for effective health care[9,10].

1.2 Concept of Culture

In the interpretation of linguistics related to the word culture, the basic meaning of the word agriculture is observed. It is suggested that the word "culture" comes from the word "Ederecultura", which is used in Latin for farming, mowing, etc.[11]. Similarly, another study suggests that the origin

6   Bayık Temel, A. (2008). Multicultural nursing education. *Journal of Anatolia Nursing and Health Sciences*, 11(2), 92–101.

7   Koçak, Y., & Terzi, E. (2012). Migration in Turkey, effects and solutions of those who migrate to urban. *Kafkas University Journal of Economics and Administrative Sciences*, 3(3), 163–184

8   Papadopoulos, I., & Lees, S. (2002). Developing culturally competent researchers. *Journal of Advanced Nursing*, 37(3), 258–264.

9   Jeffreys, M. R. (2000). Development and psychometric evaluation of the transcultural self-efficacy tool: a synthesis of findings. *Journal of Transcultural Nursing*, 11(2), 127–136.

10 Öztürk, E., & Öztaş, D. (2012). Transcultural nursing. *Batman University Journal of Life Sciences*, 1(1), 293–300.

11 Demirkan, E. (2007). *Effects of Cultural Differences on Organizational Communication in Multinational Enterprises*. Istanbul Yıldız Technical University

of the word culture is "Cultura", derived from the root of "co-" which contains meanings such as "residence, cultivate and protect" in Latin[12]. The term "Ekin", which is used as a term for culture in Turkish, is also derived from the verbs, given that the plants grown under various conditions are called culture plants. The word "culture" means that the root of agriculture is influenced by other meanings and uses that are then loaded[13].

Philosophers, educational scientists, social scientists and anthropologists are the leading researchers who produce various definitions on the concept of culture[14]. Culture in these areas, "Social heritage, the way of life, thought systems, values, etc." were tried to be explained in the angles. Previously, the definitions of "the culture of anything" have been replaced by the primary culture-oriented definition of the 18th century. In these definitions, culture was first considered as a form of general thought, and later expressed the development of social intellectuals, and was thought to be the general structure of art, and in the end of this century as "the way of thinking and spiritual life", defined in [12,13,15].

When the literature is examined, the concept of "culture", which is seen to have a large number of recognitions, has gained a new dimension today with the framework of post modernism and globalization Conceptually, in order to define culture, it is necessary to recognize and understand the practices of beliefs, feelings, thoughts, life forms, etc., which are transmitted from generations to generation, in the framework of the historical process. In conjunction with the conditions brought by globalization, no cultural structure is living in a completely separate way from other cultural groups This is precisely why it is not easy to define the concept of culture and the processes that are related to it nowadays[16]. According to Williams (2016),

---

12 Williams, R. (2016). *Key Words: Culture and Society Vocabulary* (6th ed.). Istanbul: Sena Ofset.

13 Doğan, Ö. (2012). *Cultural Sciences and Cultural Philosophy* (6th ed.). Istanbul: Notos Book.

14 Oğuz, E. S. (2011). The concept of culture in social sciences. *Journal of Hacettepe University Faculty of Polite Letters*, 28(2), 123–139.

15 Burke, P. (2006). *Cultural History* (2nd ed.). İstanbul: İstanbul Bilgi University Publications.

16 Limon, B. (2012). The Concepts of popular culture and kıtsch ın the process of cultural change. Journal of İdil, 1(3), 106–115.

the lack of consensus on the concept of culture suggests that the word stems from the use of different thought systems[17].

The concept of culture for the first time in 1871 by Edward Tylor in the book "Primitive Culture" is a complex whole that encompasses the knowledge, art, morality, traditions and other similar talents and habits that mankind has gained as a member of the Society. "described[18,19]. In this definition, Taylor combines the complex integrity of culture with his human-synthesized observation, expressing that culture has gained an abstract concept and a theory value beyond a complete definition [20]. One of the first definitions of the concept of culture belongs to Geert Hofstede. The Hofstede culture describes "the whole of a human community, which distinguishes it from the rest and the mental programs that are unique to every human community."

According to Hofstede, culture, which is a kind of mental programming process, begins primarily in the family of the individual, develops in education and working environment and continues to be added to social life. Thus, culture is transferred to the generation of generations at the end of a learning process[21]. According to Güvenç, culture, "as a member of the Society, living, by doing, learned and taught by the material spiritual is the whole complex of everything" [22]. According to the Turkish language institution, culture, "Historically, all the material and spiritual values created in the process of social development, and the creation of them, to the next generations used to convey, the measure of sovereignty of man's natural and social environment is the whole of vehicles" [23]. According to the cultural definition of the UNESCO World Cultural Policy Conference in the conclusion Declaration, culture is the widest meaning; "It is a combination

17 Williams, R. (2016).pp.24.
18 İbid., Aksoy, Z. (2013). p. 22
19 İbid., Doğan, Ö. (2012).p.18
20 İbid., Oğuz,E.S.(2011).PP.123-139
21 İbid.,Demirkan, E. (2007). P.29
22 Güvenç, B. (2015). The abc of the Culture (7th ed.). İstanbul: Yapı Kredi
    Publications.
23 TDK. (2018). Turkish Language Institution General Turkish Dictionary.

of the distinctive material, spiritual, intellectual and emotional traits that define a society or a social group, and not only in science and literature, but also in the forms of life, fundamental rights of man, value judgments, It is a phenomenon that encompasses its traditions and beliefs"[24].

To summarize the culture in the light of the definitions in the literature, "It can be said that individuals or societies are a complex whole of tangible and abstract elements that they make to accomplish their objectives in the historical process." In other words, culture is one of our vital functions. Because human beings have been trying to understand, explain and systematically question their relationship with the world since its existence, and they need to be enriched by both culture and culture by transferring it from generations to generation.

1.3 Properties of Culture

In line with the various definitions of culture, Göçer (2013) has outlined the characteristics of the culture in a more descriptive and systematic way to support culture definitions as follows[25]:

i. Since culture is a learned phenomenon, it is necessary to comply with the rules of education and the laws.

ii. The culture continues to exist between generations because it can be transferred from generation through language.

iii. The internal dynamics and teachings of each culture vary from community to society.

iv. While culture is a growing concept in social life, individual attitudes, values and behaviors also have an important place in the cultural phenomenon.

v. Culture is a dynamic phenomenon that includes private and life experiences and meets social needs.

---

24 UNESCO. (1982). *World Conference on Cultural Policies Final Report*. Mexico City. Retrieved from (Date of access:18.01.2019).

25 Göçer, A. (2013). The views of Turkish teacher candidates on language culture: A phenomenological research. *Journal of Erzincan University Faculty of Education*, 15(2), 25–38.

vi. The culture also has the power of the parser as well as the unifying. Cultures in harmony in the social arena are in a tendency to integrate.

vii. Culture is an abstract concept[26,27].

1.4 Culture's Elements

There are fundamental elements in the country or on international platforms that are common to every culture. In every society, the severity, form and nature of these elements may vary, but generally it is assumed to apply to every culture[28]. The basic elements of the culture are as follows:

i. Material culture elements: they are the material values of a society.

ii. Language: the fundamental element of communication and the most important carrier of culture.

iii. Religion and belief systems: the values in which people understand the situations they are in and the way they behave.

iv. Attitudes, values and norms: the most important factor separating the cultures from each other and determining them is the rules and values.

v. Art and Aesthetics: each culture has its own unique aesthetic perception and values.

vi. Social and political organizations: organizations that regulate the relationships of individuals in each society, shaping their social organizations such as marriage, family, education, and the organization that regulates the behavior and life forms of people within a community and Organizations.

vii. Education: in the community where the individual is socialized, the family then learns the cultural gains by training in groups of close environment, school, workplace, etc.[29,30]

---

26 İbid., Güvenç, B. (2015) p. 12.
27 Seviğ, Ü., & Tanrıverdi, G. (2014). *Intercultural Nursing*. İstanbul: Academy Publishing
28 Susar, F. A. (2005). *Evaluation of Cultural Barriers Encountered in Multicultural Environments in Terms of Public Relations and Advertising; Public Relations, Corporate Communication and Management in Multicultural Environments* (1st ed.). Istanbul: Istanbul Commerce University Publications
29 İbid., Aksoy, Z. (2013). p. 22
30 İbid., Susar, F. A. (2005). p. 13

1.5 Culture and Health

Our cultural résumé has an important role in the formation of our health beliefs, values and health behaviors. This role formats individuals "perception of health, illness and the World" [31](. The health policies of recent years in the world focus primarily on the prevention of inequalities and discrimination in health and ethnic characteristics. Therefore, studies are able to provide health care to respond to the needs of different groups of communities in cultural terms. Demographic and economic change in our multicultural world has led to the differences in the health levels of people from different cultures, health care-giving and institutions to consider cultural characteristics,[32].

Throughout the generations, human communities encountered a wide range of health problems and sought to find solutions. In all periods of history, the concepts of health and illness are defined according to cultural patterns; Mankind has struggled to treat the "disease", which is a part and a sign of life, and has made this struggle with its value judgments, beliefs, customs traditions, worldview and technology [33], [34]

Nowadays, the values, judgments, attitudes and behaviors of people, most importantly, their knowledge, are very different from the past. The people of the information age are more complex and have increased expectations due to the intensive information cycle[35]. This situation causes the concepts of health and disease to be greatly influenced by human behavior. Anthropological and ethnographic data reveals that diseases are explained in different cultures in different ways, and therefore treatment approaches differ[36,37]. This situation has revealed the concept of "health culture". Health

---

31 İbid., Bolsoy, N., & Sevil, Ü. (2006). P. 79
32 Başalan, F., Bayık, Temel,A.(2009). Cultural competence in nursing. *Journal of Social Policy Studies*, 17(17): 51–58.
33 Erci, B. (2014). *Public Health Nursing* (2). Amasya: Göktuğ Publishing.
34 Yalçıner, N., & Çam, O. (2015). The views of nurses working in psychiatry on intercultural care. *Journal of Ege University Faculty of Nursing*, 31(3), 20–36.
35 İbid., Göçer, A.. (2013). p. 27
36 Çınarlı, İ. (2016). The role of strategic-health communication in the medical health. *Journal of Communication Theory and Research*, (43).
37 Karatay, G. (2009). Kars province. identifying the practices of women living in health centers in some health-related emergency situations. *Dokuz Eylul University Electronic Journal of School of Nursing*, 1 (1), 3–16.

culture, "the ability of individuals or societies to obtain basic health services, interpret and understand information, and use these information and services for the purpose of protecting and improving health. It is also the integrity of the skills and competencies that are the product of individuals consciousness levels"[38].

The medical approach, which is in an effort to increase the expected life year with a variety of information hardware and new discoveries, ignores the need for a qualified life in which people have a say in their health,[39],[40] which hampers the will to live their realities and solve their problems. But to assimilate the perception of "healthy life" to people, the health needs to be addressed on the basis of a comprehensive cultural approach. Therefore, health must be treated as a dynamic phenomenon[41]. Health workers, who have adopted the understanding of contemporary public health and holistic approach, give opportunity to participants and have effective problem solving skills; however, it will be the product of an understanding that adopts cultural structures that give direction to values, attitudes and behaviors[42].[43].

Health and illness can affect all the balances in human life. Medically ill disease is a physiological process that manifested itself with certain symptoms, in terms of culturally individual. The loss of health and the results of the pathological process are all the perceptions of pain, discomfort, fear and pain as a result of experience by an individual[44],[45]. Therefore,

38 İbid., Göçer, A. (2013). p. 29
39 İbid.,Bolsoy,N., & Sevil,Ü. p. 82.
40 Aytaç, Ö., & Kurtdaş, M. Ç. (2015). Social origins of health-disease and health sociology. *Fırat University Journal of Social Sciences*, 25(1).
41 Tabak, S. (2002). Health Culture and Youth. 8th National Public Health Congress. Diyarbakır. Akademi Publishing, 23–28.
42 İbid., Göçer, A.. (2013). p. 29-31
43 Hotun Şahin, N., Onat Bayram, G., & Avci, D. (2009). Culture-sensitive approach: *transcultural nursing. Journal of Education and Research in Nursing* 6(1), 2–7.
44 Demirer, Y. (2006). Conceptualisation of health in the axis of culture and politics: examples of patients and diseases. *Society and Physician,* 21(1), 25–35.
45 Higginbottom, G. M. (2000). Heart health-associated health beliefs and behaviours of adolescents of African and African Caribbean descent in two cities in the United Kingdom. *Journal of Advanced Nursing*, 32(5), 1234–1242.

culture and health are largely related and each culture has its own unique health norm and approach[46]. The disease is accepted when it reaches harmony and agreement in the opinion of the people around them. "Being sick" is a social process[47]. "Perception of disease" varies according to features such as social-cultural properties, attitudes, behaviors and health service facilities [48,49]. Hence the culture is a dominant force in determining health and disease forms and behaviors[50]. Therefore, healthcare needs must be determined by making cultural assessments covering the individual's cultural heritage, health beliefs and practices[51].

Tab. 1, which is important in cultural evaluation; general questions, the individual's primary language and communication method, health and personal beliefs related to the disease, religious and family roles? Questions were included.

1.6 Evaluation Example: Wound Care

The cultural meaning of blood and secretions is assessed, and Muslims can be perceived as blood pollution. For this reason, stained bedding and clothing should be replaced immediately. Some Asians believe that blood is the life force, so the presence of bloody secretion and drainage should be explained in detail. Showing negative reactions to the individual's bloody secretions can be perceived as disrespect by some Africans.

The confidentiality of individuals in cultures that emphasizes gender-appropriate care and individual gender roles is ensured. By using bedspreads and properly covering, the body parts of the individual are prevented from

---

46 İbid.,Bayık Temel, A. (2008). p. 92-101
47 İbid.,Bolsoy,N., & Sevil,Ü. p. 82-84
48 İbid., Göçer, A.. (2013). p. 29-31
49 Birkök, M. C. (2015). Health sociological paradigms and social factors affecting health. *Turkey Clinics J Public Health Nurs-Special Topics*, 1(3), 1–6.
50 Hitchcock, J., Schuber, P., & Thomas, S. (2003). *Spiritüel and cultural perspectives, Community Health Nursing* (Pelmar Pub). USA.
51 Tanrıverdi, G.(2017). Ethnic and cultural assessment and clinical decision making. Eti Aslan, F.(Ed.), *Evaluation of Health and Clinical Decision Making* (p. 1–16) Within. Yenişehir/Ankara: Akademisyen Bookstore.

exposure. Given the maintenance of the individual's privates, it is ensured that the care giver is of the same kind.

The participation of family members is provided when explaining the maintenance application. In cultures that prefer to live in the collective, the patient waits for one of the family members at the bedside. Among Arab families, at least one family member, usually a woman, is always found at the bedside.

Different cultures give different meanings to wounds and traumas. It is important to assess and understand the different meanings about blood and wounds and how the wound affects the patient and his family. Muslims can perceive blood as dirty, so the dirty dressings and sheets should be destroyed immediately.

Dressing changes always require respect for the patient's privacy. However, in some cultures, patients may need an additional privacy; for example, if the dressings are in a private area, they can demand that the caring person be the same gender. In addition, it may be beneficial for the patient to have a family member present during the procedure. As a result, if the cultural differences considered as a wealth of life are known by health professionals, the meaning and importance of the patient to health and illness will be understood and the steps of improving health and improvement in disease are correct will be discarded. As the example suggests, cultural differences affect the healthcare processes directly. For this reason, in Turkey, which is like a Mazoaik, Balkan immigrants (Bosniak, Pomak, Albanian), Circ, Romanians and Alevi's cultural properties and their reflections on health care are addressed in this booklet.

Tab. 1: Cultural Evaluation[a,b,c]

General Questions
Where were you born?
How would you describe your cultural identity?
What cultural features are important for you?

Primary Language and Communication Method of the Individual
What language do you usually speak in your home?
How long do you judge the language spoken here (Turkish, English....)?
What language would you prefer to speak?
Do you need an interpreter?
Will you need to translate during your stay at this healthcare facility?
Is there a special ritual in communicating with your family? (for example, to whom the
questions can be routed)
Is there anything specific about your culture in oral or non-verbal communication?
Are there some symbols/signs that are indicative of respect for others?

Personal Beliefs About Health and Illness
How do you describe health and disease?
Do you believe in the necessity to control your health?
Do you have any practices and rituals that you think can improve your health?
Did you use / use alternative healing methods such as acupuncture, Ayurveda, therapeutic touch or herbal remedies?
Have you used the methods? Was it effective if you used it?
Who do you consult when you're sick?
What are the practices or rituals used to treat the health problem?
What kind of attitude do you have in mind-sickness problems?
Pain? Chronic illness? Death? Die?
Who gets health-related decisions in your family?
Would it bother you to talk about health issues?
What do you think of the inspection procedures?
How can the health team members help you?

Religious/Spiritual Influences
Do you have religious beliefs?
What are your spiritual/belief requirements?
Who do you see as a guide or support?
Do you have a belief that you feel good when you're sick?
The importance you use in events such as birth, life cycle, adolescence, marriage and death
Are there events, rituals or ceremonies?

(*continued on next page*)

Tab. 1:　Continued

What are the roles of individuals in the family? Who takes decisions in your family? Who lives at home, how many generations and people are together? What is your opinion about separation and divorce in marriage? What is the attitude and role of children in the family? How to punish children and who does? What are the major events in your family? How to celebrate? Do you have beliefs and practices related to pregnancy, birth, breastfeeding and raising children?

[a] İbid., Tanrıverdi, G.(2017).p.1–16

[b] İbid., Başalan F., & Bayık, Temel, A. (2009).p.51–58

[c] Hotun Şahin, N., Onat Bayram, G., & Avci, D. (2009).p.2–7

Do Not Forget

The most important behaviors in cultural evaluation are to be sensitive.
It should also be learned what an individual feels and what he/she believes.
Regardless of the individual's race or cultural heritage, each individual is unique.

2 Culture and Health Relationship: Turkey Rumelia-Balkan Immigrants, Romanians and Alevi Public Cultural Properties Overview

2.1 Balkan (Rumelia) Immigrants and Cultural Features

The Balkans is one of the most burned regions in the world, but still has a boiling boiler and a time bomb that is ready to explode. The Balkan Peninsula is a mountainous terrain located in the southeast of the European continent. It is named after "Balkan", which means "steep mountain covered with forest" or "mountain range" and Turkish origin. This peninsula is surrounded by the Adriatic Sea in the west, the Black Sea in the east, the Mediterranean Sea, the islands and the Sea of Marmara. The Balkans has been an area of continuous struggle due to its geopolitical-geostrategic position[52].

The migrations to Turkey are mostly due to the migration of immigrants and Muslims outside Turkey, from totalitarian regimes or from war environments to Turkey, i.e. racial, national and socio-cultural, and it is possible to indicate that it has been raised for political reasons. As a result, Turkey has been the target of "mass" migrations from surrounding regions, especially the Balkans, for over two centuries. The common characteristic of migration from neighboring countries in both the close and distant history of Anatolia is a shared culture[53]. The existence of a common cultural origin has prevented the emergence of a threatening structure that is traumatic for the norms and values of indigenous culture. However, it is still a disruptive feeling of belonging to a certain environment or culture, and for those who migrate, there can be no "what is there" and not being here. For them, past

---

52 Özcan S.(2013). *Pomak Identity*. First edition, Ceren Publishing and Bookstore, Edirne. p. 5–89.
53 Yilmaz, A. (2014). International migration: types, causes and effects. *Electronic Turkish Studies*, 9 (2).

experiences, knowledge, savings can be "usable" for the future on a line of continuity[54]. For this reason, immigrants express themselves in a number of group belonging and cultural identities, such as other social segments[55]. Therefore, immigrants attract attention because of their cultural values that they bring with them, institutionalize them and also reproduce them, and in this direction, the identity, culture, belonging and value clash, etc., are of interest. Today, immigrants from the Balkans (especially from the territories of Bulgaria, Greece and the former Yugoslavia) to Turkey have settled in almost all of the country, mainly in western Anatolia[56]. However, in order to prevent population congestion in western Anatolia, the country's general preference for Balkan/Rumelia immigrants has been the provinces in the west, although it is followed by policies that promote sedition in the central and eastern parts of Turkey. In particular, as in Bursa, Istanbul, Kocaeli, Balıkesir, Canakkale, Manisa, Edirne, Tekirdağ and Kırklareli, the city of Izmir, are the places where Balkan immigrants live in a dense area[57].

In the Balkans, there have been mass migrations to Turkey from almost every country inhabited by Turkish and Muslim countries [58]. In the literature the main common aspect of the immigration movements of the Ottoman and Republican period is that they have also been able to migrate as non-Turkish descendants. The only Republic criterion was to pay attention to the presence of non-Turkish descendants biologically and/or culturally integrated with Turks, but there was no such attention in the Ottoman

---

54 Ünal, S. (2012a). Common historical and cultural construction of identity: in Turkey, the Balkans (Rumeli) immigrants. *National Folklore*, 2012, Year 24, Issue 94

55 Çelik, C.(2003). Immigration identity between institutionalization and congregation. *Marife Scientific Accumulation*-2: 235–247

56 Ünal, S., & Demir, G. (2009). Migration, Identity and Belonging in the Context of Balkan Immigrants in Turkey. Social Transformations and Sociological Approaches, VI. National Sociological Congress, Adnan Menderes University, Aydın, 378–407.

57 Ünal, S. (2012b). The balkan (Rumelia) identity in the city of izmir as a form of social-spatial-political clustering. *Contemporary Local Governments*, 21 (3), 49–77.

58 Ozlem, K., (2011). Balkan immigrants and political elections in Turkey. www.tarihistan.org. (Accessed on 06.11.2018)

dimension.[59] Being a "Muslim" is considered as "direct and independent criteria" in the Ottoman period migrations and "indirect and dependent criteria" in the Republican period migrations. However, the predominantly common nature of immigrants of both periods was to be a Turkish descendant or to be affiliated with Turkish culture. Today in Turkey "Muhacir" as defined who Balkans / Rumelia are immigrants. These migrants are the Muslim communities who were settled in the Balkans before the Ottoman Empire and the Turks migrated back to Anatolia and who knew themselves Turkish or who had historical, cultural and religious ties with the Turks.[60]. Especially Bosniak, Albanian and Pomak culture are some of the most noticeable groups from these communities[61].

2.1.1 Pomak Culture

Pomaks general definition: "Pomak" speaking, slavic-rooted and spread to the five countries of the Balkans (Bulgaria-Greece-Turkey-Macedonia-Albania), a minority that has mostly accepted Islam, the non-Muslim Pomaks orthodox, the people who are Christians. As a legacy of the complexity of the Balkan history, there is a consensus that the pois can be a definite and reconcilement origin, although different views are defended, but they are slavic-rooted. After the Ottoman-Russian war, Pomaks came to the settlement areas within the borders of Turkey.

2.1.1.1 Pomaklar with Ethnic Properties and Population Distribution

Pomaks are described as Bulgarian-speaking Muslims residing mainly in the south of Bulgaria and in the Rhodope mountain valleys to the north of Greece[62]. The meaning of the name Pomak was first found in some

---

59 Özdal B. (2018). An international migration and population movement in the context of Turkey. DORA Printing. Company.Bursa /Turkey. 1st Edition,xii + 368. https://www.academia.edu/37994515/CUMHUR%C4%B0YET_D%C3%96N EM%C4%B0NDE_BALKANLAR_DAN_T%C3%9CRK%C4%B0YE_YE_Y %C3%96NEL%C4%B0K_G%C3%96%C3%87_HAREKETLER%C4%B0

60 Sait, R.(2010).Association and Balkan immigrants in Turkey. http://www. gazeteyenigun.com.tr. 2010.

61 İbid., Özdal B. (2018).p.12

62 .Balikci, A. (2007). Visual ethnography among the Balkan Pomak. *Visual Anthropology Review*, 23(1), 92–96.

interpretations of F. Kanitz in 1882. According to him, Pomak said that the word "pomoçi", which means "help" of the Slavon, was "Pomaçi", meaning "sidekick" and that they received the name because they saw the task of helping the Pomaks in Turkish armies [63,64]. Pomak Turks, Kuman (Kipchak) descended from the descendants of the Bulgarian and Greek for more than a hundred years, although they expressed their own national identities as the Turkish stated. The Pomaks in the Rhodopes are neighbors with the Yörükler which we know as Bozok and Çepni. It is seen that the Pomaks are affected by the Âhîlik organization which operates among Turks.[65]

No Pomak actually sees himself as a Greek. Despite all linguistic relationships, no one wants to be Bulgarian. Sometimes they claim to be Turks, but that's what they mean by the Muslims. Because during the Ottoman period, they accelerated their transition to Islam, and the cultural interaction was very much as they embraced their religion, and they felt like Turks, meaning that they were influenced and accepted from their religion from the Islamic . When asked for identities, Pomaks usually stop.

On the Pomaks, especially Bulgaria approached and sought to bulgarize them with a strict identification point of view. The Pomaks who migrated to Turkey has experienced the characteristics of the flexible identity and has accelerated their adaptation to Turkey in Turkish and has already been in religious terms and in the historical process since the Ottoman and even most Pomak itself Turkish, the effect of religion here is very large[66]. Pomaks, who are referred to different nations with different names living in five different countries of the Balkans, are not dependent on the Bulgarian, Greek, Macedonian, or Serbs, but by saying that they feel belonging to the Turks, they have seen the greatest. Despite the oppression and persecution of the Turks because of their identity by combining their identities, the motherland

63 Memişoğlu, H. (2005) *Pomak Folk Songs in the Balkans*. Istanbul: Turkish World Research Foundation.

64 Alp, İ. (2012). *The Turks of Pomak* (Kumanlar And Kipchaks). Edirne: Trakya University Publications.

65 Http://www.Turkcebilgi.Com/Ansiklopedi/Pomaklar (Date of access:14.11.2018)

66 Öztürk, N., & Aşçıkoca, H. (2013) Environmental, spatial - programmatic and structural evaluation on the houses of Osmaniye town of Pomak. International Journal of Social Research, 6(25), 410–428.

they have taken refuge in Turkey, and therefore the name of the Turks as well as the traditions brought by the identity of Pomak.

The Pomaks are in groups, with high plateaus and plains separating the Meric plains from the Aegean shores, and they live in the Green Valley Rhodopes of the Karasu (Mesta) rivers and in the regions of Pirin and Vardar Macedonians. Pomaks have settled in various regions of Anatolia and have come to these days by continuing to live their own cultures and reconfiguring a culture of synthesis. In Turkey, Pomaks is heavily inhabited in Balikesir, Kırklareli, Tekirdag, Edirne, Bursa, Çanakkale, Eskişehir, Izmir, Manisa and small groups in Samsun, Kütahya, Afyon, Konya and Niğde. Around 3 million Pomak lives in the world. An average number of more than one million in the Balkans and a few million Pomak masses in Tur key[67,68,69,70]

2.1.1.2 Pomaks with Religions and Languages

The most abused subject language is used in the Pomaks. The language in which the Pomaks speak varies according to the country and region where they live. Pomaks are living in Bulgaria and speaks a language close to Bulgarians. Looking at the Pomaks that are living in Macedonia, they speak a language similar to the official Macedonian. However, 30 % of the language that the Poms speak was found to be Ukrainian Slavonic, 25 % Nogayca, 10 % in Arabic words. The slavic word in Pomak dialect is quite high. Ten percent of Arabic is due to the fact that the Pomaks are Muslim[71,72].

---

67 Erdinç, D. (2002), The economic situation of the Turkish minority in Bulgaria in the change process, the Turkish encyclopedia, Ankara: Turkey Recent Publications, 20, (394-400)

68 Dürük, E. F. (2007). *The pesne practice in Pomaks: symbolic culture and ethnicity* (Unpublished PhD Thesis). İzmir: Dokuz Eylül University Institute of Fine Arts.

69 http://pomaknews.com/pomashkiselo (Date of access 16.11.2018)

70 Eroğlu, M. A. (2015). Balıkesir sındırgı (sahınkaya vıllage) the pomak weavıng. *Journal of İdil Art and Language*, 4(18), 185-204.

71 İbid.,Memişoğlu, H.(2005). p. 94.

72 Dzhuvalekov, S. (2011). Religious Life of Pomaks (Doctoral dissertation, Selcuk University Institute of Social Sciences).

Pomak, the language spoken by Pomaks, is accepted as one of the mouths of southern Slavic language. Although in time, not as a scientific goal, but for political purposes, the language of the is considered to be a mouth of the Bulgarian or ancient Greek origin, but there is not enough detailed research on the Pomace language. However, the research suggests that the grammatical and the sentence are of Slavic language. In the Balkans and Turkey, the language has not been developed due to the lack of educational language, and the separation of other Slavic languages in the Balkans has deepened. It is easier to write with Cyrillic alphabet. The equivalents of sounds such as ya-TS-ch cannot usually be expressed in Latin with a single letter. There are five known poems[73,74,75]. They are:

i. **Pomak of Lofça Region**
ii. **Pomak of Rhodope Region**
iii. **Pomak of Western Thrace Region**
iv. **Pomak of the Drama, Karacaova and Tikveş Regions**
v. 5-Pomak of Gora (Albania)[76,77].

Pomak language 70 % and higher rates salvia, maybe around 20 % Turkish (in many states in the Balkans, the Turkish word rate is close to this ratio, from living in the Ottoman administration for many centuries) and in smaller proportions and the region consists of other languages and dialects.

In reality, no Pomak sees himself as a Greek. Despite all linguistic relationships, no one wants to be Bulgarian. Sometimes they claim to be Turks, but that's what they mean by the Muslims. Because during the Ottoman period, they accelerated their transition to Islam, and the cultural interaction was very much as they embraced their religion, and they felt like Turks, meaning that they were influenced and accepted from their religion,

---

73 http://pomak.blogspot.com/.(Date of access 16.11.2018).
74 http://pomaktarihi.blogspot.com/2011/04/pomaklar-uzerine-dusunceler1.html (Date of access 16.11.2018).
75 Günsen, A. (2013). Pomaks as a Balkan community and evidence of Turkishness in their perceptions of identity. *Journal of Balkan Research Institute*, 2 (1), 35.
76 İbid.,Memişoğlu, H.(2005). p. 94.
77 İbid., Dzhuvalekov, S. (2011). p.22

"Islamic."[78] More than ethnic identity in the Pomaks, religious identity is prominent. They qualify themselves as Muslims. After Islam, ethnic identity is held in second degree. Old Pomaks do not qualify themselves as Turks or Bulgarians. They call themselves just Pomak. However, nowadays, the new generation of young people accept themselves as Bulgarians. The Bulgarian state is trying to separate the Pomaks (Muslims) from the Turks. Whereas Islam is the common point that joins these two ethnic groups. Most of the Pomaks are Muslims and are dependent on the Hanafi sect. It is noteworthy that the old religions of shamanism have taken care of the traditions of the past before the Islamism[79].

2.1.1.3 Marriage and Family Structure

In the Pomaks, the family union has a dominant structure for men. Large and huge family is common. This aspect coincides with the family structures of the Central Asian Turks, especially the Kazakh family structure. In Anatolia, the father's authority and respect for the traditional family structure is extremely strong[80].

In the Pomaks, it is very common to marry with the method of kidnapping, which is common in Anatolian and Central Asian Turks, although the rate is gradually falling. The kidnapping was a ritual necessary for the legitimacy of marriage until recently in Altay and Ruby Turks. The kidnapping of girls in the Turkish communities in Central Asia and Anatolia is a tradition of indulge when it occurs in the meaning of marriage. Although it is banned in the cosways, it is a form of marriage that is of found today ,[81]. In addition, it is stated that leviratus-style marriage was applied in the past. In this kind of marriage, a brother with a wife and older brother or younger brother can marry. Likewise, this form of marriage is a kind of

---

78 http://pomaktarihi.blogspot.com/2007/04/kaypedilen-kimlikpomaklar.html .(Date of accessed: 16.11.2018).
79 İbid., Özcan S. (2013) pp.5-89.
80 Taşdelen, M. (2008). *Onn the Customs of the Gorillas: The First Determinations, Rock Gora Monument at the Top of the Hill*, Editor: Ebubekir Sofuoğlu, Istanbul: Fsf Print Hause. 11–25.
81 Kalafat, Yaşar (2006). *The Turkish Folk Beliefs from the Balkans to Ulugh Turkestan, Ankara.*

marriage that is seen both in Anatolia and in Central Asia. In the Kazakh people, when the husbands of young and beautiful women died, the woman did not return to her parents' house if she was widowed, she became a wife to her deceased brother or younger brother or a close male relative. At present, the realization of marriage among families with a relative distance of seven umbilical distances has been determined. This form of marriage (Eczogami) is also valid in Kazakh, Kyrgyya, Bashwolves, Altaylar, Yakut, Uyghans, and other Turkish communities outside of Oguz Turks. The interesting thing is that the Turks in the Balkans are also Anatolian, but they do not approve of a related marriage[82].

2.1.1.4 Approach of Health and Disease

85–90 % of the Pomaks that have a significant resemblance to the traditions of Anatolia in their socio-cultural life are living in villages and dealing with agriculture. Home furnishing and women's clothing are very similar to the style of upholstery clothing of Anatolian villagers.

In the obscure periods of ancient times, the belief of Pomak ancestors' gaze into the world" was basically divided into two parts. The parts that cover the goodness, the beauties, and the parts where the feeling of gratitude is ceremonied, and the evil, the diseases, the absence, the inefficiencies, the infertility, the sections they believe are dominated. They care about the protection of the evil and the opposite behaviors and the deliberately opposing ceremonies to ensure efficiency in production, and magic were used as an important counteract. These rituals will occasionally be referred to as the "people who seek immortality in the Balkans" by their sister peoples. In the face of dangers filled with natural phenomena bearing grasping Pomak human instincts with a great moral support for the negative nature of the phenomena that he described as evil against the sorcery, hoping for a little bit of magic tomorrow. In order to be more assured, he was able to transfer all the things that he had made to the next year through traditions while waiting for the miracle of his rituals. In these days, Bocuk's mother's, Bocuk's wife's, Bocuk's grandfather's names are celebrated by the Sedenka and Pomaks. Despite this cultural ritual, festivities, spells, magic

---

82 İbid., Özcan S. (2013) . pp.5-89.

and abundance are intertwined. The night of the winter was the starting symbol of the nights that were the hardest in the evening[83]. If the water freezes these nights, it is believed that the year will pass in abundance and blessings. In most Pomak villages, the "Bocuk boar" statement for very fat people is still widely used, and it is a reference to a healthier growing of the pig in the cold. The people of Pomak, after 1870 genocide and migrations with other Muslims in their new dormitories in the Marmara and other Pomak settlements in Thrace where they brought together they still continue their customs.

The newborn child is given a tip to the first news. The baby is first washed with salt water and is given to the spouse to celebrate the birth. The Macedonian pogs call this tradition "Babina" and other Pogs "Smidal/ Simidal". The main goal is to feed the bread soaked in sugar, which is called Smidal, as well as meat dishes. The baby is attached to the evil eye. It is important for children to remove their first teeth and to give gifts to those who inform them. The "tooth" is arranged to celebrate the emergence of the first tooth. It is believed that the women who have had a new birth are haunted by the "Al Karısı", "The Nightmare", and "Al-Basma", the evil spirits called by the people. For the protection of these evil spirits, a red belt is attached to the waist of women who have had a new birth for 40 days. The tradition of connecting the red cloth to brides seen in shaman culture is similar to this tradition of Pomaks.

As in the Turkish artillery of Anatolia and Central Asia, the grandfather of the house, which is the largest in naming the child, takes precedence. In this practice, every family has to know the names of seven belly-horses. This is also true in kazakhses and other Central Asian communities. Turkish names such as Arslan, Demir and Turan are given. The presence of these names evokes the idea that they remain in balance from the pre-Islam period.[84,85,86,87]

---

83 http://pomaknews.com/?p=8057(Date of accessed: 16.11.2018).
84 İbid.,Taşdelen, M. (2008). Pp. 11–25.
85 İbid., Kalafat, Yaşar (2006) . pp.5-89.
86 İbid., Özcan S. (2013) . pp.5-89.
87 Çetin, N.(2011). The ottoman census in the subdistrict of tiryanda - çengele village in 1905 (1321 in islamic calendar), (Date Access:14.11.2018).

In some Pomak communities, women don't do handicrafts on Thursday night and Friday. If done, the young children who die, the ibriks are drilled when they carry water to the parents, so they have faith that they cannot deliver water Tuesdays and Fridays are not cleaned and laundry is not washed. On Tuesdays, the nails are not cut. In other days, the cut nails are buried in the ground. It is believed that it will be unlucky if not done[88].

2.2 Culture of Albanian

The Albanian community has been in the 15th period following the Byzantine rule. He lived under the Ottoman rule for nearly four centuries and 80 % of Muslims became an independent state in 1912. Therefore, it is a European society, but it has largely adopted Islamic values during the Ottoman period. After independence, it was ruled by the kingdom until the Second World War, and the interaction with European relations and Western culture in this period gained intensity[89].

2.2.1 Albanians with Ethnic Properties, Population, Languages and Beliefs

Albanians are one of the oldest and most settled nations in the Balkans. Albanians, who are based on the ancient Illyrian's live in Albania, Kosovo, Macedonia, Montenegro, Greece, Turkey and many European countries. Their population is estimated to be around 9 million. Albanians, who are rooted in culture and traditions, have been involved with more Turks, Greeks, Italians, Russians, Germans and Serbs in the history[90]. In the framework of these relationships, the changes in religion, language and culture of Albanians have occurred. The historical Albanian culture, based on the Ilıyrian has preserved many traces of it in the past, although the Albanian culture, which has been familiar with Roman, Slav, Ottoman culture and

http://acikerisim.deu.edu.tr/xmlui/bitstream/handle/20.500.12397/5045/Necat. pdf?sequence=1&isAllowed=y,

88 İbid., Özcan S. (2013) . pp.5-89.

89 Saygılı, H. (2014) 20. Starting from the Ottoman and Perception of Turkey in today's Albanians century. *Wise Strategy*, 6 (10).

90 Azimli, M. (2006). *Albanian grand vizier husband (dervish) davut pasha, international albanian among the six centuries*, Pristina, Kosovo.

Communist cultures, has protected itself against them. However, Islam and Christianity religions and secular and capitalist Western culture have an important place in the formation of the present Albanian culture.[91] After the Balkan wars, Albania, termed Ilıyria, was torn apart. After the breakup, Albanians were divided into three, Albania, Macedonia and Kosovo Albanians. Albanians, who were separated after the split, began living with Macedonians, Serbs and Bosnians in their region and began to break down from their own cultures[92].

A very important feature of Albanian culture is the tolerance that is shown between religions. This value has existed since ancient times. In Albania, there are many different religions, such as Bektaşi and Sunni Muslims, Orthodox and Catholic Christians and Jews, who have lived together and are still living. Throughout history, there has been no religious distinction between Albanians. The most important factor for the stability of the separation was marriages between religions. Therefore, there are many Albanian families who have different religions and parents. In Albanian society, these values have held a crucial place until the Second World War[93].

Albanian: Indo-European languages. Linguists also find Albanian close to the Baltic-Slavic (East), Indo-European and Germanic (North) languages. In the course of years, the words taken from other languages did not affect the language in terms of grammar and phonology.[94].

2.2.2 Marriage and Family Structure

In Albania, the family constitutes the foundation of society and families have many children. They have embraced living in the large family model,

---

91 Shehu, F. (2011). The influence of Islam on Albanian culture. *Journal of Islam in Asia* (E-ISSN: 2289–8077), *8*, 389–408.

92 Zhelyazkova, A. (2000). *Albaniam dentities*. Albania and the Albaniam dentities. Edited by antonina zhelyazkova. Sofia: International center for minority studies, Pp. 9–63.8, September 2006, Priştina, Kosova

93 Likaj, M. (2013). A study of the perception of social value of Albanian youth. *Süleyman Demirel University Faculty of Arts and Sciences Journal of Social Sciences, 29*.

94 http://www.nkfu.com/arnavutluk-dini-ve-dili-hakkinda-bilgi/

far from the core family structure. The oldest man establishes the authority of the family, and the thought of the outback is taken by his own decision, leaving the administration of the house to the other "oldest man". The woman in the family is very valuable, and in the absence of a man, the house is said: "Albanian families valued women very much, and they counted it with great force. Marriages are also made between family agreements. It is also noted that the marrying people are of the same life level. The nest is dominated by strict discipline and is given importance to the family. The head of the family is not a tyrant, but a master of the house. There is a democratic order in the family, decisions are jointly taken [95].

Family bond are very reputation so that Muslims get Christians and never have marriages between residents of the same village. The administrative authority of a local region is the oldest member of the most important family in the region. The woman who is attached to her husband in the family is free in public life, and does not hesitate to tell her opinion in both family matters and in the country. It is also an intriguing point for the woman to boast of her own beauty and dignity, rather than her own children and their talents. The mother of many children sees great reputation in society. The inability of the woman to be seen with her partner in social life or even in the war farewell is a concern that increases her dignity more than restricting her freedom. Despite all these privileges, the Albanian woman will never appear among the people with her husband. They will succeed her husband in the war. However, if the country is in danger, it is women who stand up and raise the men first to intervene or revolt[96].

2.2.3 Approach of Health and Disease

As in the Turks living in various geography of the world, Albanians from Turkish groups in the Balkans also have many beliefs and practices related to birth, pre, order and after. The menstrual and application of birth is also ongoing today. Birth is always regarded as a happy event for a family. It is a

---

95 http://www.arnavut.com/mizac-ve-aile-yapisi//(Date of accessed. 16.12.2018).
96 Doğan, A. & Garan, B. (2013). *The Memories Are Reflected in Albania and Albania*. VIII. International Congress of the Grand Turkic Language, Albania Tirana, p. 427–451.

miracle that increases the respect and affection of parents and fathers in the family and in society. The status of woman and man with birth varies. The dignity of the community increases. There has been a similarity in the value given to the mother in societies that have been closely related to Turkish society and Turks. Motherhood, which has been given to the woman who is born, has provided the woman with respect and protection[97].

The couple's own decision to make children across Albanians. The delayed status of pregnancy is normally met, and in ancient times, the women who were barren were despised and gossiped by Albanians, and rumors were done, and a variety of applications were made for the elimination of infertility, the child in Albanians Women are taken to old women and their bellies are made by different applications through sieves. According to this belief, the woman's abdomen is collected and fulfilled. Besides sieve, pottery is used for the same process. In addition, I hope to be creative in infertility, teachers or shrines and candles are burned and the Quran is distributed in 1 night, the Hatim is read. The boy's face is like a piece of moon, looking at beautiful people, and judging by the ugly, his child is believed to be ugly. To determine gender, they throw a pinch of salt down the head without your mother knowing, if she scratches her head, she scratches her back, the male, the pregnant woman touches her nose first, the boy is believed to have the girl if she touches her mouth. If the mother is beautiful during the pregnancy, the boy will be the interpretation of the girl, if it gets ugly. The woman's abdomen is cheesecloth to avoid miscarriages. If the child is reborn in the dice, the dice will not be discarded until the child grows. The application of opening the window is also done to make the birth easy. When the milk of the woman who gave birth is reduced, the syrup is smoked, milk and sorbet

The things that evoke death are sickness, seeing babies born in the dream, the rooster of the night singing, the constant barking of dogs, in the window or close to the owl singing, the bride in the dream to see the Aunt (wedding), the patient wants me to go to say, it's like seeing teeth in a dream,

---

97 Koca, K. S. (2018). Common cultural elements seen in the transitional periods of the Turkish-Macedonian-Albanian-Bosnian communities in Macedonia. *International Journal of Turkish Literature Culture Education*, 7 (2), 1085–1103.

seeing someone naked, etc. It is not uncommon for people to make negative comments about dreams[98] .

2.3 Culture of Bosniaks

2.3.1 Ethnic Characteristics, Populations, Languages and Their Beliefs of Bosnians

The Muslim public who maintains their presence in the Balkan geography and speaks slavic is called Bosnian. Bosnians, mostly from Bosnia and Herzegovina, Serbia and Montenegro, are related to the Serb and Croat communities, other Slavic-rooted societies of this geography. The main issue separating Serbs, Croats and Bosnians from each other speaking the different mouths of the same language living in the same geography is the difference in religion and sectarian. The cultural differentiation of these three societies; It is determined that Croat is Catholic and that Serbian are Orthodox and Bosnian Muslims ,[99] The Catholic Croat on the Balkan Peninsula is next to the orthodox Serbian identity; Muslim Bosnians are the result of the Ottoman Empire's conquest of the region. A significant part of Bosnia and Herzegovina was conquered by Fatih Sultan Mehmet in 1463. The socio-cultural result of conquest outcomes and the influence of Turkish Dervishes settled in the region, the crowds became Muslims. With the adoption of Islam in Bosnia and Herzegovina, changes in socio-cultural aspects have begun to be seen. The concepts of new religion and the way of life, the institutions (madrasas-Lodges et al.) felt in Bosnia and Herzegovina; the major cities of the region such as Sarajevo, Banja Luka, Travnik, Mostar have won the appearance of a classical Ottoman city with its social structure. With this change in the social structure, the ancient influence of Ottoman Turkish was seen in the Balkan Slaved (Bosnian, Serbian, Croatian). Turkish words, expression, mold words used in daily life. This situation is reflected in the literary texts. A century after the Ottoman Empire left the region, the quantity and functionality of the Turkish language in the Bosnian (Serbian and Croatian) is due to the effect of Ottoman Turkish in the Balkan lang

---

98 İbid., Doğan, A. & Garan, B. (2013)., p. 427–451.

99 Eker, S. (2006). On ethno-linguistic structure and Turkish language and culture in Bosnia, *National Folklore*, 72 (18), 71–84.

uages.[100,101,102] The Balkan Peninsula is one of the world's most recognized language science districts. The Balkan language science region is located in 6 Slavic languages (Serbian, Croatian, Bosnian, Montenegrin, Macedonian, Bulgarian), 1 Latin language (Romanian), independent Greek, Albanian and non-Indo-European language, Turkish. One of the most important characteristics of the relations between these languages is the linguistic phenomena that arise as a result of the contact with the Turkish language. Dialects of the border lines in the Balkans are seen[103].

Believe in Allah: there is no problem in the faith of the boss to Allah. They all believe in God. They have a belief in God, as they hear from their fathers, their mothers. The respect of the Holy Quran is like the respect of the Muslims of today's Turkey in the Qur'an. The religious beliefs of Bosnians pushed them into wrong practices. The belief that all evil and good deeds will be seen in the afterlife has pushed Bosnians not to seek their rights. Instead of eliminating him against any injustice that comes to their heads, it is a very common belief that Allah does nothing in the afterlife. Faith in fate is parallelization with the beliefs of the afterlife. They accept everything that comes to their heads by saying that we are destined to live a life that is indexed to fate. Hajj worship is a worship made by Bosnians who have come to a certain age, as in Turkey[104].

2.3.2 Marriage and Family in Bosnians

It is a kinship that Bosnians are most meticulous about marriage. The Bosnians, who are very sensitive about this, are very careful not to be related to anyone who is married. Those who do not comply with this situation

---

100 Malcolm, N. (2002). *Bosnia a Short history*. London: Panbook.
101 İyiyol, F. (2010). Traces of the Turkish-Tekke Sufism in Bosnian Folk Culture. Unpublished PhD Thesis, Sakarya: Sakarya University, Institute of Social Sciences.
102 Nurkić, K. (2007). *Islamization process in Bosnia and Herzegovina*. Unpublished Master Thesis, Samsun: Ondokuz Mayis University, Institute of Social Sciences.
103 İbid., Eker, S. (2006). Pp.71–84.
104 Tacoğlu, T. P., Arikan, G., & Sağir, A. (2012). Migration and cultural identity in Bosnian immigrants: the example of Fevziye village. *Electronic Turkish Studies*, 7(1).pp. 1941–1965.

are condemned by the Bosnian community. The form of marriage we call Exogamy is common. It used to be the family type, the family head, the wife, married sons, brides and the traditional large family type where single children lived together. In addition, the traditional family was smaller than the large, and the family chief's own parent was seen as the temporary family type where his single siblings lived together. But nowadays, with the change of conditions, large families are torn apart and left to the core families, which is the general state of today's Bosnian families. Whether it be in the traditional family or in the temporary family or in the core family, promises and domination are in the father.[105]

2.3.3 Approach to Health

The child is one of the most important enrapture that increases joy and happiness, as in all societies in Bosnian. This situation is much more important for the mother because a woman without a child is likened to a fruit-free tree in Bosnian society and is not deemed acceptable. In this context, as soon as the baby comes into the world, it is welcomed by all family members because it saves the mother from a difficult situation. A gift, called the Gospel Gift, is dealt with close relatives and the subject of the neighbor's grandparents or any other elder. Two or three days later, the child is made to name a ceremony. This ceremony is an appropriate ceremony for the Muslim tradition[106]

Bosnians are to be protected from diseases, to get rid of themselves of troublemakers, and to protect the evil eye from the amulet. When they do that, they believe they'll relax. Reading by whoever: They go to teachers to avoid diseases such as the Amulet and the evil eye. They prefer to read more than go to the doctor. To shed a bullet: to understand the cause when something comes to their heads, and to eliminate this trouble, a job that Bosnians do is to shed a bullet [107].

---

105 Demir, G., & Bolat, S. (2017). Identity and belonging in Circassians. Journal of Sociological Studies Conferences, (55).pp.1-42.

106 Tacoğlu, T. P., Arikan, G., & Sağir, A. (2012).pp. 1941–1965.

107 Aslan, C. (2005). *Circassians in the Eastern Mediterranean, Adana,* Caucasian Cultural Association Publications. p. 1–186

2.4 Culture of Circassian

2.4.1 The Distribution of Ethnic Properties, Religion, Language and Population of Circassians

Circassians are Caucasian immigrants who have migrated to Anatolia in various waves since 1880. In particular, some of the Caucasian immigrants who left their lands in 1864 with the pressures of the Tsarist Russia took refuge in the Balkans. After the 93, a group that lived in the Balkans emigrated to the Ottoman territories. The Ottoman Empire placed immigrants in masses by developing a settlement policy. According to the Ottoman settlement policy, Circassians were placed on the Anatolian and Rumelia banners, the Black Sea coast and the large areas of the region such as Konya, Sivas, in connection with the ability to create a buffer mechanism[108]. Circassians are the people of the North Caucasus Mountains, autochthonous (which have been built since the present)[109]. The word Circassian is not only used to refer to the same ethnic origin. Circassians are defined as the names given to all peoples from the Caucasus. It is also known as a people originating from the contact of the Greeks culture of a part of Asia Minor or migrating from the Arabian peninsula. Although the Circassians are the people of the North Caucasus, the numbers in the North Caucasus today are quite small. As a result of the pressure policies applied by Russian executives, Circassians were forced into exile. Nowadays, Turkey, Syria, Jordan, Palestine, Egypt, Yugoslavia, some European countries and the United States, Canada, such as the lives of many different countries. It is also in the sources that the word circa (Kerketai), which comes from ancient Greece, has been changed to the present day. In the literature, it is stated that the word Jarkaz, which is known as the minds of the people in the North Caucasus, is transformed into circatic or circa in the Turkish language in time, which means that it operates in the fields of Tatar

Circassian settlements in Turkey, around 600, are scattered all over Anatolia except Thrace, eastern and southeastern regions. The busiest Circassian settlement is located in Sinop, Samsun, Çorum, Amasya, Tokat,

---

108 Namitok, A. (2003), Çerkeslerin kökeni (Çev. A. Çeviker), Ankara, Kaf-Dav Yayınları.
109 Papşu, M. (2004 Mart), Anadolu'daki Abhazya, Atlas, Sayı:132, 118–131.

Yozgat, Sivas, Kayseri, K. Maras, Adana, Middle western Anatolia and Marmara region (Eskişehir, Bilecik, Bursa, Balıkesir, Canakkale, Yalova, Sakarya, Düzce). The Circassian population in Turkey is estimated to be between 2 and 3 million. Circassians 19. At the beginning of the century, they were separated into the subgroups of Cemguy, bje, Jane, Hatukay, mapleasing, Mambeğ, Abzeh, Şapshallow, Natuhay, Ademiy, Yegerukay, Nutriey, Kabardey and Ubıh. At the end of the war and exile some disappeared or confused others. Some researchers count a separate ethnic group based on their own language. Circassians are Sunni Muslims; from the 16th century, they embraced Islam through Ottoman and Crimea Turks. Their language was named Cirali, and later this term was used only for North Western Caucasian languages, and its use in recent years has been limited to only include"Adigece" [110].

Today, the settlements of Circassian cities are Sakarya, Düzce, Bilecik, Hendek, Inegol, Bursa, Izmit and Eskişehir. There is also the line of Samsun, Tokat, Yozgat, Kayseri and Adana from the North Caucasus where the Cirkaans from the Karatay-Çerkez region settled. The two regions in Samsun and Eskişehir are mixed with the [82.83]. Circassians are a relatively late Muslim society. 16.–17. Since centuries, they have become Muslims through Ottoman Turks and Crimean Tatars. Apart from a Christian community of 3,000 people living in the Mozdok region of North Ossetia in the Caucasus, all of the circles are Muslims[111]

2.4.2 Marriage and Family Structure

In Circassian families, marriage institution and domestic relations have significant differences, except for similarities with the Turkish family structure. For example, "The new bride does not speak to the father-in-law and his wife's elderly relatives. It appeals to his wife and all of his relatives, not by name, but by pseudonym. It's kind of rude for your father to show close attention to his wife and children. Women participate in all social events not with their wives, but with other brides of the family or with neighboring women. Similarly, this situation is seen in the Turkish family structure.

---

110 İbid., Nurkić, K. (2007). *p*.27-36
111 Demir, G., & Bolat, S. (2017). p. 55.

However, with the change of urbanization and socio-economic environment, the change of family relations can be observed in both cultures. There is a large family and kinship relationship in Circassians. Relatives determine the general social structure. This structure is determined by the relations between individuals and families, the settlement forms, the rules of marriage, the position of the woman. People are surrounded by a relatives of 40–50 people with close relatives [112]. Marriage in Circassians is a serious and somewhat problematic issue. Because of the concept of broad kinship, marriage is forbidden even with distant relatives, the same village is not welcome to choose a spouse. It is also noted that in the case of marriage, the peerage, which is the origin of Circassian, is considered to be a divorce in circasis and marriage is not very welcome, monogamy . The essence of Circassian family life is "formal" in terms of seriousness. Everyone knows their place; Neither shallow patriarchal nor artificial matriarchal rules dominate[113].

2.4.3 Approach to Health

Traditional Circassian cuisine, which is not too much to be used for bread and vegetables, is very rich in grain products, boiled/dried and meat dishes. Dairy products such as Circassia cheese and kefir also hold an important place in this kitchen. Circassian Women don't drop babies if they're murdered, and they don't prevent pregnancy. In the process of pregnancy, women do very mild work in order to give healthy birth, and have little sexual intercourse. A gift is given to the woman who gives birth, donuts/pies, Aries/lamb, etc. They give great importance to clean, healthy growth and good education of the children they bring to the world. For example, the baby is washed twice-three times in the morning and in the evening [114]

112 Aslan, C., Sefer E. B., & M Papşu. (2011). Biz Çerkesler, Kafkas Dernekleri Federasyonu, Ankara, http://www.circassian.us/Makaleler/Biz-Cerkesler.pdf. (Date of access 21.12.2018)

113 Yildiz, Y. (2018). Notes on the Circassian culture in the works of the 17th and 18th century Westerners. *Abant İzzett Baysal University Journal of the Institute of Social Sciences*. Volume: 18, Year: 18, Number: 1, 18: 219–240.

114 Kalaycı, İ. (2015). Circassia (Circassians) in terms of history, culture and economics. *Eurasian Studies*, 47(1), 71–111.

2.5 Culture of Roman

The Romans, which they live in with their peculiar culture and personality traits, and even those who are approached by prejudice by other minorities, intimidation, oppression, assimilation, severe penalties and murder in the western territories in which they migrate over time has a history of dating. In our age, Roma are faced with social policies that are produced with an approach that will involve themselves with their culture and needs.

Considering the ethnic groups that are living in Turkey, one of the examples that can be given to the concept of "prominent other" is the Roman that feel its presence in almost every region. Everyday life habits, preferences for physical appearance and their specific behavior, as well as Roman. Socio-economic and socio-cultural properties are also a different ethnic group to be easily noticed in social life. The Roman, commonly referred to as ley gypsies , are a marginal group of disadvantaged groups within the social and political spheres of interest as well as their employment, economic activities, their position in education and employment processes in urban and rural areas. The Roma, who migrated to the Anatolian geography around the 10th century, have been an inseparable part of society since then with their cultures and extraordinary lives[115,116].

2.5.1 Romans with Ethnic Properties, Populations, Languages and Beliefs

The origins of Roma, whose origins have long been discussed, have been identified as North West India.[117]. This is detected, 18. Towards the end of the century, it emerged as a result of studies made by the languages of the Roma and especially the work done by Hungarian scientists.[118] The origins of the Roma in Turkey, the Byzantine era "Atsinganoi (Athinganoi)"

115 Arayıcı A. (2008). *Stateless People of Europe: Gypsies*. First Edition. Istanbul. Kalkedon Publications.

116 Ünaldı, H. (2012). Living a cultural change in Turkey: gypsies, *Batman University Journal of Life Science*, 1 (1): 615–626.

117 İbid., Kalaycı, İ. (2015). Pp.71–111.

118 Kurtuluş, B. (2012). *Gypsies as a Stateless People: Their Origins, Problems, Organizations, (Der.)* Levent Ürer, Being Roman, Gypsy Stay, Istanbul: Melek Publications: 17–43.

which is known as witchcraft/fortune telling astrology, rituals and Christian dualism as worship of a different form of the present Eskişehir. It is stated that it is based on a group of Refrigerans who lived in the area around[119]. Their homeland is 9 and 10. In the case of abandonment in the centuries, the Roma have entered Afghanistan, Iran, Anatolia and the Balkans as the first arm. They came to Anatolia about 10th century. As the second arm, Roma in Afghanistan, Iran, Armenia, Russia and the Balkans; the third arm is 15. With the century, they moved through Afghanistan, Iran, Syria, Palestine, North Africa and Spain into various countries of Europe [120].

"Dom" and "Lom" from two different linguistic novels of India origin, the domes are mainly in the Middle East and North Africa, and the Lomas reside in eastern Anatolia and the Caucasus. The first relations of the Roma with the Turkish society are based on the Seljuk Turks. The first dates of arrival in Istanbul were determined as 1050. The Roman population of Modern Turkey is composed of three main linguistic groups, the Roms, Doms and Loms. The Roma have sub-identities such as bushes, mangos, Gevende, Karachi and Mıtrip, but their identities are permeable.

The mobility of Roma in terms of professional or local groups ensures that these borders are permeable and loose [121]. The Roma, which are called by different names in different geographies because they have a nomadic culture, are 18. In Eastern Europe in the century, "Kalderspouse" was referred to as "Gatinos" in northern Europe. Since they came from Egypt, they were called "Gypsy" by the British and French. Romanians living in Romania; "Ramon", the inhabitants of Hungary, "Çigan", the people living in Spain; "Phiamanko", the people who lived in Germany are named as "Mohem" or "Romani". One of the other groups is known "Kıptî" [122]. Romanians called "Tsigani" in Croatian, "Sigan" in Kyrgyz, are named "Çingane" in Farsi[123]. In addition to these naming, Roma can be referred to differently

---

119 Marsh, A. (2008). *Ethnicity and identity: the origin of gypsies*, (Jun.) Ebru Uzpeder, Savel Danova/Roussinova, Love Ozcelik, Sinan Gokcen, (trans.) Ezgi Taboğlu and Sezin Oney We are here!: Roma in Turkey, Discriminatory Practices and Rights Struggle, Istanbul: March Printing: 5–27.

120 İbid., Kalaycı, İ. (2015). Pp.71–111.

121 İbid., Ünaldı, H. (2012) .pp.615-626.

122 İbid., Arayıcı A. (2008). p.12

123 Mezarcıoğlu, A. (2010) *The Book of Gypsies, Istanbul: Cinius Publishing.*

even in regions within a country. One of the most frequently used names in western Anatolia and Thrace, the Roma, referred to as the "romen ", has many names in other parts of Turkey. For example, the Roma, referred to as "the Elekçi" in the Mediterranean and Aegean regions in Central Anatolia are referred to as "Mutrib" in the vicinity of Van and Ardahan, "Cano" in Adana, Erzurum, Artvin, Erzincan, Bayburt and Sivas as "Poşa". In many provinces of Anatolia, they are commonly referred to as "Coachman"[124]. The name "Brunette citizen" is used in various geographies as a more general description . When asked whether they describe themselves as Roman or Gypsy, the participants who live in Turkey responded as "of course Roman"[125]. However, it is also stated that it should be made a neutral word using the word "Gypsy", which is free from the negative meanings it contains[126].

Looking at the distributions of Roma in the world; According to the population estimates, the number of Roma in the world is approximately 30 to 40 million. Romania is the center of Roma population in Europe, and Roma are about 10 % of the country's population. Bulgaria, Spain, Hungary, Slovakia, Turkey, the former Yugoslavia and the Czech Republic, after Romania, are the countries where Roma have the most inhabitants, respectively. Researchers and activists in Roma and non-governmental organizations (CSO) suggest that the Roma population in Turkey is between 2 and 5 million[127].

According to Marsh (2008), Turkish gypsies are divided into three basic groups Dom, Lom and Rom in the language context. The Doms, which is a branch of the Dom Chinese in the Middle East, live in the eastern and southeastern regions of Turkey and usually plays drums-zurna and earn their lives . This community, also known as the Kurdish gypsies, is called Mutrip by local people, and is named Karachi, but they define themselves

---

124 Kolukırık, S(2009) *Gypsies from past to present: cultural identity language history istanbul: Ozan Yayıncılık.* p. 59.
125 Yanıkdağ, T. (2012). *Türkiye'de yaşayan romanların sorunları genel bir bakış,* (Der.) Levent Ürer, Roman Olup Çingene Kalmak, İstanbul: Melek Yayınları: 247–270.
126 Aksu, M. (2003). *Türkiye'de çingene olmak.* 2. Baskı, İstanbul: Kesit Yayınları.s.50.
127 İbid., Ünaldı, H. (2012).pp. 615-626.

as Dom [128] and although Kurmanci, Zazaki and Turkish speak, they protect the Domari dialect [129]. The Lomas, which are located in the northeast of the country through the Caucasus, are referred to locally as Posha and speak the language of Lomavre under the influence of Armenians. The romlar, which forms the third arm of the migration wave, is composed of communities with Romanes dialects, which are transferred to Europe and Western Anatolia through Russia and the Balkans [130]. The country where the Roma live is stated that they adapt to the region and even the cultural structure and the religion and language of that region [131].

According to the status of Roma citizens living in Turkey in employment, it is seen that those who are employed in permanent jobs among the Roma and who have social security opportunities are very few. The unskilled jobs that Roma citizens can find are generally concentrated in areas based on the elimination of. It is expressed by the Roma citizens that they are very concerned about the area where employers are residing in recruitment. Roma offers an employment opportunity for people who hide from the citizens of the real identities of racism and intolerance against the income of seasonal labor Roma citizens in Turkey [132]. The work of Roma citizens in practice, in order to sort jobs on a sectoral basis, shoe painting, Porter, old item collecting, basket-shop, flower-dealing, peddling, bundlilism, garbage collector, back material aggregator for conversion, bear player until 1995 is prohibited, fortune-teller in touristic centers, trade, horse-riding, carriage driving, charioteers, musician, performer, dancer, puppetry, storytelling and fairy tales, basket knitting, knife making, metal processing, are in place. The decrease in demand for some professions such as basketwork, the occupation, and the elector has caused the loss of these professions [133]. They have

---

128 Önder, Ö. (2009). *Gypsies*. K. Emiroglu, and S. Aydin. in the Dictionary of Anthropology (pp. 196–201). Ankara: Science and Art Publications
129 İbid.,Ünaldı, H. (2012) pp.615-626.
130 İbid., Yanıkdağ, T. (2012) pp.247-270
131 İbid.,Yıldız, Y. (2018). pp.219-240
132 İbid.,Ünaldı, H. (2012) pp.615-626.
133 Özdemir, A. (2014) *Working in Roma: poverty, sample of Sakarya Gazipaşa neighborhood*, Master Thesis, Sakarya University, Social Sciences Institute, Sakarya.

been busy with temporary jobs that are flexible and not tidy because they love to live free, and others do not want to work at your disposal. In this context, the traditional professions that they pursue have been active in their cultural survival. Although the literature is aware of the importance of education, it is emphasized that the education cannot continue due to exclusion and financial opportunities.[134] In his study, Kolukırık (2006) stated that the level of education among Roma was low[135]. In the study results abroad, it is noted that the education level of the novels is low.[136] In all countries where Roma live, there is even a problem of lack of education in different regions of the country[137].

2.5.2 Marriage Pattern and Family Structure

In their ability to sustain the traditions and professions of the Roma, there is also the share of Endogamy (inner marriage) preferences. For Roma, their children are the goal and essence of their lives. Because the children of the Roma have been working in the built-in life, they do not bring an economic burden.[138] Looking at the activities of Roma citizens living in Turkey. They do not link their activism to minority rights or other identity-based efforts[139]. Marriage is an exception among Romans, but marriages occur between Romans . In the literature, the Romans of Edirne are also closed

---

134 Tanriverdi, G., Ünüvar, R., Yalçın, M., Acar, P., Yaman, B., Akçay, E., ... Sürer, M. (2012). Evaluate Gypsies' Living in Çanakkale According to "Purnell' Cultural Competence Model" *Journal of Anatolia Nursing and Health Sciences, 15(4).243–253.*

135 İbid., Kolukırık, S(2009) p. 59.

136 Campayo JG, Alda M.*(2007).* Illness behaviors and cultural characteristics of the gypsy population in spain. *Actas Espanolas Psiquiatria 2007; 35(1):59–66.*

137 İbid., Kalaycı, İ. (2015). Pp.71-111.

138 Genç, Y., Taylan, H. H. & Barış, İ. (2015). The role of social exclusion in the educational process and academic achievement of Roma children. *The Journal of Academic Social Science Studies, 33: 79–97.*

139 Gökçen, S. ve Öney, S. (2008). In Turkey, Roma and Nationalism (Jun.) Ebru Uzpeder, Savel Danova/Roussinova, Love Ozcelik, Sinan Gokcen, (trans.) Ezgi Taboğlu and Sezin Oney, We Are Here!: Roma in Turkey, Discriminatory Practices and Rights Struggle, Istanbul: March Printing: 129–135.

to marriage and social relations with non-Roman[140]. Kolukırık (2006) in his study between the Izmir gypsies determined that Gypsies were not warmly looked after their relatives[141]. It was also emphasized in the literature that the family chief of the Roma was a man, that women participated in domestic decisions, but the decision mechanism played a dominant role in the man, respected the elderly, and that monogamy was widespread[142]. Ozkan (2006) in the study of the age of marriage for women in the 13–17, Roma for men has determined as 15–19[143]. According to the results of a study conducted in the Spanish Roma, early marriage and adolescent maternal mothers were widely identified. The literature points out that Roma women are 30 years old and grandparents are 35 years old[144].

2.5.3 Approach to Health and Disease

The cultural characteristics of the Romans differ with the society they live in. Recognition of these cultural features is important for the acceptability of health care. In the countries where Roman live, it is seen that they are more exposed to behaviors that negatively affect health than other groups. In health care, Roman citizens living in Turkey, the refusal of their treatment, the sloppy attitudes encountered in hospitals, the material burden of drug costs and therefore the arbitrary implementation of the treatments have indicated that they are suffering from the issues[145]. However, difficulties in accessing the personal documents required for formal transactions may also prevent them from occasional health and other fundamental rights and services[146].

---

140 Ceyhan, S. (2003). A case study of Gypsy/Roma identity construction in Edirne. *Unpublished Master's Thesis. Ankara*: Middle East Technical University, Institute of Social Sciences. 147–154
141 İbid., Kolukırık, S(2009) p. 59.
142 İbid.,Özdemir, A. (2014) p.31
143 Özkan AR.(2006). Marriage among the Gypsies of Turkey. *The Social Science Journal*. 43(3): 461–470.
144 İbid., Kurtuluş, B. (2012) *pp*.17-43.
145 Cleemput PV, Parry G. Health status of Gypsy travellers. *Journal of Public Health Medicine*. 2001; 23(2): 129–134.
146 İbid.,Ünaldı, H. (2012) pp.615-626.

The health problems between Romans are similar from past to present and continue[147]. Early marriages between Romans, adolescent pregnancies, substance abuse, infant and child deaths, difficulties brought by nomadic lives, inability to have hygiene conditions, inadequate and unbalanced nutrition, unprotected sexual intercourse, unwillingness to use condom[148,149], heart diseases, diabetes, hypertension,[150] high incidence of infectious diseases, limited use of health care resources, lack of communication with healthcare workers ,[151] and many negative behaviors affecting health are more common than other groups[152].

In the study of Sutherland (1992), it has determined that heart, diabetes and hypertension are common among Romans. Romans said that the use of alcohol and smoking among men is widespread [153]. The use of cigarettes among Roman women was widespread[154]. The literature states that the Romans applied to the traditional practice. Reasons for application include economic insufficiency, inability to reach healthcare, lack of education, dissatisfaction from health care[155].

147 Molnár Á, Balazs A, Antova T, Bosak L, Dimitrov P, Mileva H, Pekarcikova J et al. Health impact assessment of Roma housing policies in Central and Eastern Europe: a comparative analysis. *Environmental İmpact Assesment Review.* 2012;33(1):7–14
148 Kabakchieva E, Amirkhanian YA, Kelly JA, McAuliffe TL, Vassileva S. High levels of sexual HIV/STD risk behaviors among Roma (Gypsy) men in Bulgaria: pattern and predictors of risk in a representative community sample. *International Journal of STD & AIDS* 2002; 13(3): 184–191
149 Kelly J. A., Amirkhanian Y. A., Kabakchieva E., Csepe P., Seal D. W., Antonova R, Mihayiov A, Gyukits G. Gender roles and HIV sexual risk vulnerability of Roma (gypsies) men nd woman in Bulgaria and Hungary; an etnographic study. *AIDS Care* 2004; 16(2): 231–245.
150 Sutherland A.(1992). Cross-cultural medicine. A decade later. *Gypsies and Health Care.* West J Med 157(3): 276–280.
151 Campayo JG, Alda M. Illness behaviors and cultural characteristics of the gypsy population in spain. *Actas Espanolas Psiquiatria* 2007; 35(1): 59–66.
152 İbid., Ceyhan, S. (2003). Pp.147-54
153 Molnár Á, Balazs A, Antova T, Bosak L, Dimitrov P, Mileva H, Pekarcikova J et al. (2012). Pp.7-14
154 İbid., Önder, Ö. (2009).*pp.*. 196-201.
155 Özyazıcıoğlu N, Öncel S. *Cultural Approaches in Child Care. Intercultural Nursing.* First Edition. Istanbul. İstanbul Medical. 2011: 203–239.

Arayıcı (2008) has stated that the Roma are living in the suburbs and slums in general, which are not suitable for health[156]. According to the study conducted in the UK about Romans the health status of the novels was found worse than the worst of the British population socio-economic level.[157] Berberoğlu, et al. (2001) in their study in Edirne, the Roma have determined that they know and use the healthcare facilities largely. The reason for this is that the economic level is low and the prevalence of green card usage is shown[158]. In a study comparing the lives of Roma in different European countries, it is noted that Roma live in areas with poor physical living conditions in general[159].

2.6 Culture of Alevi

2.6.1 Alevis with Ethnic Properties, Populations, Languages and Beliefs

Alevism: It is an Islamic belief formed by the interaction of motifs belonging to different religions and beliefs in Anatolia with some motifs belonging to Islam[160]. The origin of the word Alevi is Arabic, meaning "belonging to Ali" and "belongs to Ali". The plural form of the word Alevi is Alevîyye and Alevîyyûn. The word of flame according to the denominational and Sufi conception is, "to count and depend on Saint Ali." Therefore, the term "Alevi" can be used for anyone who loves, counts and depends on Saint Ali. It was also used to signify the meaning of the Alevi of Saint Ali, as well as the belief system of political, mysticism and

---

156 İbid.,Arayıcı A. (2008). Pp.22
157 Cleemput PV, Parry G. Health status of Gypsy travellers. *Journal of Public Health Medicine*. 2001; 23(2): 129–134.
158 Berberoğlu U, Eskiocak M, Ekukulu G, Saltık A. The use of novels and others in primary health care center in Edirne province. *Society and Physician*. 2001; 16(6): 470–475.
159 İbid.,Özkan AR.(2006). pp-70.
160 Yazıcı, M. (2011). *The Understanding of Alevism: Sociological Analysis of the Alevi Sayings and Gülbangs in Kavalcık*. Unpublished PhD Thesis. Firat University, Institute of Social Sciences, Elazığ.

objection[161,162]. The fact that the philosophy of a Alevism of life is also seen as a religious structuring, which means that Saint Ali is a follower[163,164,165]. The Alevi's are not only in Turkey, but also in terms of ethnic beliefs and cultural values that can be found outside the geography of Turkey. The elements of Alevi belief and culture have been an integral part of Anatolian culture throughout history. The Alevism is the product of a broad period of time extending from the 10th century to the present day and a wide geography from Central Asia to the Balkans[166]. Alevi's culture is mostly on oral tradition. Oral tradition is also one of the sources of Alevi culture. However, with the influence of modern culture, there is a rapid development and change process. Identifying and recording elements of Alevi culture in such a process seems to be a serious necessity.

The vast majority of the Alevi's of the Alevi community, which began at the end of the 1950 and in the 1960, showed a huge increase in the rural areas. This migration also allowed the Alevi's to benefit more from social mobilization. However, it has also caused the settlement of the village communities which constitute the basis of immigration worship and is based on oral culture, and the Alevi of the people with whom there is no institutionalization is cut or distributed along with the migration to the city[167]. With the migration from the countryside to the city, the socio-economic structure in the community, socio-spatial patterns, social relations and roles, beliefs

---

161 Dalkıran S. (2002). An experiment on the Alevi identity and the Anatolian flame. EKEV *Academy of Journal*, 6 (10), 95–118.

162 Üçer C. (2005 a). Worship life in traditional Alevism and the approaches of the Alevi to basic Islamic prayer. *Journal of Neuroscience Academic Research*, 5(3), 161–189.

163 Gümüş N. (2011). *Women in Alevism: The Perception of the Women in the Şahkulu Sultan Dervish*. Unpublished Master's Thesis. Dumlupınar University, Institute of Social Sciences, Kütahya.

164 Özcan A. K. (2013). A field study on the Muslims of Alevis. *Tunceli University Journal of Social Sciences*, 2 (3), 27–44.

165 Taşğın A. (2009). Cem, Cemevi and Functions. Alevi-Bektashi Culture from Past to Present. (Ed): Ahmet Yasar January. Ankara: Ministry of Culture and Tourism Publications. 211–225.

166 İbid.,Üçer C. (2005a). pp.161-189

167 Şahin B. (2015). Alevi Identity and Revolt Teaching. *Journal of International Social Research*, 8(39), 539–548.

and cultural institutions, such as a radical change in the situation to cope with the traumatic effects of[168].

Even if a sizeable part of the Alevi's lived in Istanbul for many years, they came from geography such as Turkmenistan, Khorasan, Uzbekistan, Iran, etc. The phenomenon of immigration brought about the phenomenon of unemployment, as well as in general the religious elements are shaped [169]. There are various discussions and definitions of the origin of Alevism. The Alevi's are differentiated by ethnic, political and religious according to ethnic differentiation, in Anatolia, Turkish, Kurdish, Arab, Turkmen, Kurdish flames in the Zazalar, the Mediterranean and some of the Aegean, "Tahtacılar", the Black Sea, "Çepniler", domestic Anatolia, "Abdallar" different Alevi's communities. In the form of buying another hand, the flames are ethnic origin: (a) Turkish/Turkmen origins (b) Kurdish origins (c) Zaza origins (d) Arab origins (E) Albanian roots (f) The origins of the Persian (g) or classes of other origins.[170]

Turkish Alevi's are not very strong in economic care. Most of the Alevi's migrated to Istanbul in the years 1980–1990 and after 1990 and are composed of economically weak community members. A group that aims to live in urban culture and has relations with more educated and political parties constitutes the wealthy ones of this community.[171] A large part of the Alevi's that have migrated to Istanbul and found a place in urban life are very poor in terms of economic conditions, the economic opportunities brought by urban culture, cultural events and some social services, They live their lives with little or no benefit. This is a cause that reveals or nourishes the "urban tensions" in urban space at times. In the upper income group of the Alevi's: those who are considered to be rich constitute about 5 %, whereas a 20 % slice accepts themselves in the lower income group, which

---

168 Salman C. (2017). Turkey location of the flame experience in migration and urbanization: a periodization proposal. *Journal of Faculty of Economics and Administrative Sciences, (Special Issue),* 24–51.

169 İbid.,Gümüş N. (2011). p.30

170 Gezik E. (2013). *Alevi Kurds: religious, ethnic and political issues.* Istanbul: Communication Publications. 1–27.

171 Aktaş A. (1999a). Changes in the family structure in the transformation process of the rural. *Turkish Culture and Journal of Hacı Bektaş Veli Research,*12, 1–60.

is more evident in the imbalance in Turkey's income distribution. It shows that we are also in Alevi's. The Alevi's that assess themselves economically change their political preferences and the understanding of social justice in the lower income group, which is effective in the form of different demands of the flames[172].

There is a significant difference between the Alevi economy and other economies. In the culture of Alevism, the production is dependent on the requirement and this is a production based on the nature conditions. Production in other economies is essential. It is calculated that the needs of the Alevi are determined and divided into the production. In the study, the Department of Labor can participate in the work and they are evaluated as a whole and are calculated over the balance of the Labor Department calendar, the workforce ones and the non-potential. There is no profit in flame, unjust gain and no provision. Professional production and training are kept alive as master-apprentice relationship. Production is made in mind of the poor and the helpless. Consumption is divided into bites[173].

2.6.2 Religious and Language Features

Because the essence of faith in Allah is the common denominator of all Muslims, a person who does not believe in Allah is not considered a Muslim. Therefore, it is not possible to have such a Alevi. There is no hesitation in the Alevism of Allah at the point of faith[174]. The adoption of the Gog-Muhammad-Ali is often used in both the need of everyday life and in the practices of the rights, the belief of the amalgamate; Saint Muhammad was the last representative of the Prophet's light, namely, the prophethood of; Saint Ali represents the understanding of custody[175]. In his Alevism conception, four great books are believed and there is no negative reference to the Qur'an [176]. In the structure of Alevism, the belief of the afterlife in

172 İbid.,Şahin B. (2015). Pp.539-548.
173 http://hasanharmanci.blogcu.com/hizir-Alevî-ekonomi-politigi/20418896 (Date of access:15.06.2018).
174 Yeşilyurt T. (2003), Faith dimension of Alevi-Bektashism, Islamiyat *VI*, 3, 13–30.
175 Bulut H. İ ve Çetin M. (2011). Religious beliefs and experiences of. e-Makalat *Journal of Sectional Research,3*(2), 165.
176 İbid.,Dalkıran S. (2002). Pp. 95-118.

cultural sources "mead" in a field research conducted together with some of the Alevi's "life after death by entering another mold of the human soul" is defined as a reincarnation Interpretation of the understanding of the[177]. It does not deny certain prayers in Alevism as ordered in the Qur'an. In fact, some Alevism perform prayer and fasting as in the Sunnis or reduce the prayer to three times. They pray to the public in the worship of the Alevi and the fasting prayer, as in the Sunni, is not a fasting held during the month of Ramadan, but there are fasting for certain days. Therefore, they are separated from the Sunni with the form of the application of the Alevism of the Alevi. The Alevism of worship, the shapes and the time are not in the form of certain worshippers, they accept and apply the secret relationship between God and man.[178] Consequently, the principle of "*the idea of unity*" and "*having the hand, waist and tongue*" constitutes a system of principles describing the style of Alevi thinking. The idea of unity is "*faith in God*" is the fundamental rule, however, "*joining Cem*", "*Semah*", "*Niyaz*", "*taking hands from the grandfathers/dads*", "*Hizir fasting*", "*Muharrem fasting*", and "*the end of Muharram fasting*", "*Report*" A wide range of applications such as "*Holding Musahip*", and "*Hakkullah/Giving Çıralık*" are included.[179]

As a ritual language in the Alevi society, it mainly uses only Turkish language. The subject of communication is shaped under two different headings and the communication is shaped accordingly. The first is the communication with different individuals and other societies that are not Alevi, and the second is the communication in the Alevi society that the individuals have established with each other. When communicating with different societies, they use Turkish effectively, and they know the Kurdish

---

177 Üçer C. (2005b). *Traditional Alevism in Tokat*. Ankara: Ankara School Publications.

178 Şahin M. (2011). Concept of community and family in Alevi tradition. *Journal of Kalam Research*, 9(1), 263–284.

179 Aktaş A. (1999b). *The sociological evaluation of the incidence of flames in urban environment and the frequency of applying belief rituals*. Ankara: Gazi University Turkish Culture and Hacı Bektaş Parent Research Center Publication. 449–482.

language at least at the level of comprehension. This indicates that flames do not have any difficulties communicating with different societies[180]. Alevism are used for dialect according to their culture and ethnic origin. Kurdish Alevism refer to themselves as Kırmanc and dialects as Kırmanckî. Dersim-Tunceli, Erzincan, Sivas, Muş, Erzurum, Alevi Kurds talk about my lecture. Zazas, who are Alevi, speak of Kırdaski/Kırdaşki dialect[181]. Arab Alevi's speak Syriac/Lebanese dialects. The older generation still speaks Arabic while the younger generation speaks Turkish. A large majority of the Turkmen of Turkmen origin speaks the Turkmen dialect of Oghuz Turkish [182]. Alevi society does not make the gender distinction in patriarchal structure which is valid in a large part of Turkish society in social communication among themselves, there is a greeting The Alevi community generally prefers to remain silent at times of sadness, fear, anxiety and loud voice in times of illness[183]. (There is no obstacle to eye contact or touch while telling love. The gender gap in general is not a communication barrier. In a study, the characteristics of health in Alevi society, the level of consciousness in health and their perspective toward health workers are parallel to the general characteristics of Turkish society and it is seen as important. Positive attitudes towards health care workers [184].

Alevism society does not make the gender distinction in patriarchal structure which is also valid for a large part of Turkish society in social communication among themselves. Especially in terms of health, gender is not any communication barrier for communication among individuals. There is a distance based on respect with healthcare workers. The fact that the mother tongue is Turkish prevents the difficulty of communicating with the health worker. Health workers, nurses and doctors, especially in Alevi society is seen as important and valuable professional workers. Healthcare

---

180 Çınar F., ve Eti Aslan F. (2018). Evaluation of Anatolian Alevi people living in Istanbul with "Purnell' Cultural Competence Model" *Journal of Human Sciences, 15*(1), 98–111.

181 Keskin M. (2003). The beliefs and rituals related to death in the flames of the Sarısaltık quarry (Tunceli Karacaköy Example). *Erciyes University Journal of Social Sciences Institute, 1*(15), 115–130.

182 İbid.,Üçer C. (2005b).p.21

183 İbid.i Bulut H. İ ve Çetin M. (2011). P.165.

184 İbid., Bulut H. İ ve Çetin M. (2011). p.165

workers are not only those who care for diseases, but also as people whom they entrust their lives to, and do not value superstition as an alternative to medicine because they entrust their lives to them. Male and female guests can easily share the same place within the house[185].

2.6.3 Family Structure and Marriage

Although the distribution of the head of the family and the roles in the household seems to be similar to the patriarchal Turkish family structure, it is seen that gender equality is more important in Alevi society. Family structure is suitable for traditional Turkish family. It is seen that the mother and father usually stay with the youngest child, while the head of the family is the one who produces or brings home bread. Core family structure is not as dominant as other communities [186]. The origin of Alevism also has an ancient and feminine belief, nourished from a matriarchal society. Alevism, women and men are created equal, not the sex of the souls, not the body, the soul is important, the woman has a structure of thought that is not defined by gender and honor, worship by both sexes. Aktaş (1999a) found that 83 % of the family structure in the Alevi villages were core, 12 % were traditional wide, 3 % were temporary, and 2 % were fragmented families. It is often emphasized that the nuclear family is most general [187]. However, data on family types of Alevism are not sufficient in the data of TUIK[188].

The continuity of family life and family institution is very important in Alevi and Bektashi society. Young people are encouraged to marry, and marriage is recommended. Marriage in the Anatolian Alevism. It is accepted as the circumcision of Muhammad. If a man and a girl like each other and decide to join their lives, they will be chopped off after they are gathered in the presence of Alevi grandfather. This marriage is a religious marriage[189].

---

185 http://hasanharmanci.blogcu.com/hizir-Alevî-ekonomi-politigi/20418896 (Date access:15.06.2018).
186 İbid.,Bulut H. İ ve Çetin M. (2011)p., 165
187 İbid., Aktaş A. (1999a). Pp.1-60
188 Yalçın H. (2016). Child rearing and position of women in Alevi culture. Turkish Culture and *Journal of Hacı Bektaş Veli Research*, 79, 79–94.
189 Rençber Fevzi (2012) The historical origin of the "Cem House" in the Alevi tradition. *Journal of Religious Studies, 12*(3), 73–86.

Marriage in Alevism is done in the marriage apartments based on the norms of the modern legal system[190]. The Alevism, like Hz. Ali, he has a family structure that defends monogamy. Even if it is known that Islam was allowed up to 4 wives in Islam, the Alevi faith was accepted as the only one from the old Turkish faith. In Alevi society, polygamy is not accepted and is not tolerated. Divorce without a valid reason or for no reason, the Alevi community treats the divorced party in accordance with the principles of social deprivation and declares that it does not approve the work done. In order for the request for divorce to be accepted, it is necessary that there should be negative behaviors that can never be accepted by the Alevi community, such as being unfaithful to any of the spouses, excessive misunderstanding between couples, unjustified slanders, using the right to eat and manslaughter. There is no valid reason for divorce in these cases and they are not accepted . It is difficult to talk about an exclusivist approach to women in social life within the Alevi faith. In some cases, women have a more important function than men with the identity of Fatma Ana. The idea that men and women have an equal place among Alevism who continue the tradition still maintains its effectiveness[191]. The treatment of women in the Alevism and the woman is not miserable is a commandment order. This is also the necessity of the Turkish ceremony. The woman must also be respectful to her husband. The family has a bond of mutual love and respect. Woman counting man is one of the basic conditions[192]. Marriage in Alevism and Bektashism is a blessed phenomenon. In marriage, both sexes contract and contract to live together and they live together. According to the principles of the Alevi faith, it is so important to be faithful to the word given should be kept for life[193]. According to the Bektashi belief that a man can divorce

190 Albayrak A ve Çapcıoğlu İ. (2006). Folk beliefs and practices in a middle anadolu village in the Ahl-i Sunnah tradition. *Religious Studies*, 8(24), 107–132.

191 Bahadır İ. (2005). *Women Dervishes in Alevi and Sunni Dervishes.* Istanbul: Water Publishing House.

192 Dierl A. J. (1991). *Anatolian Alevism.* (trans. Fahrettin Yiğit). Istanbul: Ant Publications. 157.

193 Menemencioğlu B. (2011). Women in Bektashi and Alevi Culture. Turkish Culture and *Journal of Hacı Bektaş Velî Research*, 60, 129–140.

his wife, first of all, it is imperative to get permission from the master (with the knowledgeable and exemplary human characteristics). Although there is a limited number of women who do not accept polygamy, there are examples of marrying. Couple marriages, the first woman is obliged to show consent . In some cases, the Alevi community is an obstacle to marriage, or even if it is shunned, it causes the marriage to be accepted as invalid. These conditions are: those who are incapable of fulfilling the role of participants, those with mental illness, minors and sex-changers. People who have sexually transmitted diseases can only get married after treatment is removed[194]. Marriage in the process of marriage in order to allow the consent of both sides is sought, otherwise the marriage is not minimized. In addition to these general rules, there are some prohibitions imposed by Alevi beliefs. For example; Mürşid-i Kamil (the person with knowledgeable and exemplary human characteristics) with the demanding (is a word used for all Alevis who are not descendants of the prophet) the Talib does not kill the mother of the murshid women or daughters. This ban is indefinite. The mourning of the priests and the relatives of the second degree until the fourth generation is not destroyed. There is no marriage between the first degree relatives of the races and their relatives up to the third generation[195,196]. The consanguineous marriage is not prohibited, but the Mut'a marriage is not a matter for Alevi[197]. Along with urbanization, a more tolerant approach to Alevi-Sunni marriages is established; Endogamy, internal marriage, understanding is effective [198,199]. In Alevi society, although gender equality is given importance, even though individuals are equal in terms of communication and social roles within the family, belief and patriarchal structure outweigh the fact that a marriage is made during the establishment of the family. One of the highlights of the transaction can be

---

194 Ünlüsoy K.(2009). An Investigation on Women in the Alevi-Bektashi Tradition., II/2,p 55–90.

195 Kaya H.(1995). The rules of Alevism. Istanbul: Engin Publishing. 39.p. 45.

196 Kaplan A (2003). Family and Kinship Institution in Aleppo, Alevism. Istanbul: Book Publishing.

197 Noyan B. (1995). Bektashism What Is Alevism? (3rd Edition). Istanbul: Ant/Can Publishing.

198 İbid.,Aktaş A. (1999b). Pp.449-482.

199 İbid., Kaya H.(1995). p. 45

done even if the consanguineous marriages, which constitute serious risks for both parents and babies, are prohibited medically, but only marriages made with people of different faiths are not welcome as a requirement of their beliefs and customs[200].

Respecting the mother and father, respecting the other family of the family, respecting the neighbor's right and the service is essential in the understanding of the family of Alevism. The most important role of the family is to ensure the continuity of the generation and to cultivate good individuals[201].

Alevism, which is a social belief institution, has an important social structure that has a system of important values and contributes to the spread of democracy and tolerance. With this social structure, respecting scientists and scientists, avoiding mistakes, loving to serve others, avoiding injustice and looking at the future, the essence of not seeing the poor and life at all times trying to gain values like society[202].

In the Alevi community living in rural areas, there were no significant changes in family relationships and roles of family members. While the man works outside the house, provides the means of living the house and regulates relationships outside the home, the woman deals with many things like domestic consumption actions, reproducing the domestic environment and maintaining good relations between the members. In Alevism, men and women respect each other[203]. Basic element in Alevism is human, gender is not important[204]. Equality between men and women is seen in every aspect of society. An example of this is that parents do not discriminate

200 Süleymanov A. (2009). Family and marital relationships in contemporary Turkish societies. *Journal of Social Policy Studies*, 17 (17).
201 http://www.sarisaltikvakfi.org/pages/article/12/Alevîlikte-aile-kavrami[Date of access: 17.06.2018].
202 Gül İ. (2014). Alevism as a social system. *Hünkâr Alevîlik Bektashism Academic Research Journal*, 1(1), 67.
203 Korkmaz E. (2008). *Anatolian Alevism, Philosophy-Faith-Doctrine-Erkanı.* Istanbul: Berfin Publications.
204 Çamuroğlu R. (2010). *Alevi revival in Turkey, contrasts.* The Alevi Identity (3rd Edition), Olsson T., Özdalga E., Raudvere C. (ed.), (Trans. Bilge Kurt Torun, Hayati Torun), Istanbul: History Foundation Yurt Publications.

between boys and girls. Male and female rights are equal in marriage[205]. In Alevi society, women have equal status as men. The woman who has a voice in the house is at the same time outside the house, not the man, but with the man.

This position in the family and the solidarity and solidarity with the man manifests itself during the implementation of the women's gender, the religious ritual for the Alevi culture and belief, and during the implementation of the necessary men. In Alevi families, it is a characteristic feature that women are valued in social life and that women are in life without being isolated from social life. Male and female guests can easily share the same place within the house. Women are considered sacred in two main characteristics of motherhood and mothers [206]. Maternity represents the productivity of women, which is an indication that the basic element in the family institution is actually female[207].

In Alevi societies, the value given to the child starts from the wedding, birth and infancy. The tradition of putting a doll as a symbol of increasing fertility in front of a bride's car in wedding ceremonies is common. Women who do not have a baby for medical reasons often apply to traditional practices. Some practices, such as amulets, places to visit, wolf pelts, and the embrace of the child in the fortune ceremony, are related to the importance given to the child. The placenta, which fulfills the vital functions of the prenatal baby, is buried in a place where the placenta will not foot in Alevi societies since it is seen as a partner with the child[208].

Traditional practices in Alevi communities in rural areas continue[209]. A boy is asked to "smoke the hearth". Girls are taught household chores from the age of 5–6. Demirbilek (2007) states that girls are not sent to

205 Gümüş N. (2011) Women in Alevism: Perception of Alevi Women in Şahkulu Sultan Dergâhı. Unpublished Master's Thesis. Dumlupınar University, Institute of Social Sciences, Kütahya...
206 Özcan H. (2005). *The value of human beings in the culture of Alevi Bektashi influencing Asian societies*. I. International Symposium of Asian Philosophical Society, Istanbul.
207 Ulusoy Y.D., Karşıcı G., ve Selçuk A. (2013). In the faith system of the Beydili Village of Sivas. *Journal of Human Sciences*, 2(2), 22–43.
208 İbid.,Albayrak A ve Çapcıoğlu İ. (2006). Pp.107-132.
209 İbid.,Gümüş N. (2011).p.34.

school after primary education[210]. However, according to the Turkish Statistical Institute, 2013/2014 period, 4 + 4 + 4 of the transition to the system, though in different classifications of this year, Turkey's overall vision of elementary education in the ratio of girls is 98,4 %[211]. The responsibility of children in the extended family does not belong to the mother who gives her birth alone. All the women in the family share the responsibility of her children. Mothers and daughters are more separated than fathers. For example, mothers have more stringent rules for eating after meals than men, not being taught after primary school, working in domestic jobs at a young age, and considering that boys are more valuable for the continuation of the lineage . However, with the migration to the city, gender discrimination in rural areas has begun to ease. Nowadays, girls' education and studies are adopted as well as boys. In the family, the woman has the right to speak. With the increase in education levels, the Alevi women in urban life enter into working life. Birth control method with urban life is on the agenda. There are fewer children. Since children are born in the nuclear family, responsibility is not a common topic of adult women in the extended family as before, but is predominantly maternal. Since the mother no longer works in the field and is in the house, the older child has avoided looking after the little brother. Families are now working for girls to read [212].

2.6.4 Approach to Health and Disease

The basic rule of being healthy in Alevism is with the environment; natural, supernatural and social relations are based on good and balanced relations. Because in the definition of health, elements such as being aware of cold-heat avoidance and knowing the small-large are important. Interdependence or imbalance in the relationship with the environment means disease. Negative

---

210 Demirbilek M. (2007). Children in Alevi Culture. *Journal of Society and Social Work, 18*(2), 65–75.
211 TÜİK- Turkey Statistical Institute (2014). *Child with Statistics*. Ankara: Turkey Statistics Institution Press, 72.
212 Güleç C. (2000). Transcultural view of health concepts in Anatolian culture. *Journal of Clinical Psychiatry*, 3 (1), 34–39.

effects of cold-heat, disbelief and lack of knowledge of the smallest plays an important role in explaining the disease[213].

Nutrition is a condition that is directly related to the economic situation or income. In this respect, the Alevi people consume, albeit at a minimum, as per the economic situation . Some foods have an important role in nutrition in Alevi and Bektashi. In particular, the salt-bread-water sanctity, the people's life in many ways entered into the food. The beliefs and practices of the Alevi and Bektashi's related to Tuzla are common. Bektashi salt is sacred. The place of salt is very important both in daily food culture and in places related to worship. It is started by tasting salt before meal and finished with salt taste. All animals that are not ruminant and double-nailed in Islam are considered as murders. Alevism do not eat rabbits. There are many reasons for this. The rabbit is menstruated and his flesh is very bloody and unhealthy. Rabbit is also an animal with its physiological and biological structure. The rabbit's head resembles to the cat's head, ears to the ewe, toes to the feet of the dog, toes to the cat feet and to the tail's tail[214]. Negative habits such as alcohol and substance use which may adversely affect health are not included in daily life [215].

In the prevention and treatment of diseases, the relations with the environment are tried to be balanced and improved. The best examples of this feature are satisfying angles, sacrifice, sacrifice, rejoice orphans, go to the dervish lodges and peace with the thugs. In the traditional health-illness system, family members, relatives and wider social groups undertake treatment, counseling and care tasks. Myths and narrations have an important place in the prevention, diagnosis and treatment of diseases, and experiences and known practices have directing and reinforcing effects .

Beliefs such as evil, evil eye, goblin, amulet and magic are beliefs that are very common in Anatolian folk culture. Considering these folk beliefs, those who do not believe in beliefs such as fortune-telling, amulets, goblin, evil eye, magic are more in Alevi society. In the production of drugs, nature,

213 İbid.,Güleç C. (2000). Pp.34–39.
214 Ergun P. (2011). Alevism on the mythological origins of rabbit belief in Bektashism. *Turkish Culture and Journal of Hacı Bektaş Veli Research*, 60, 281–306.
215 İbid.,Yalçın H. (2016). Pp., 79-94.

people, animals and plants are used. In addition, household items, clothes, sacred beings, natural beings and events are used in the treatment of magic (words or actions) [216]. Although these methods are not approved for women who do not have children, such methods as humiliation, wish-keeping, amulet, etc., these methods can be appreciated in places where modern medicine is insufficient [217].

Despite all sorts of medical developments, Alevism continue their beliefs and practices about childbirth even though they are not as vivid as they used to be. Preparations started before the birth of the baby, continue with the birth. The purpose of all these practices is to protect the mother and child from the diseases that may occur during childbirth. In the Alevism, when the first step of the new house of the bride takes her first step, a little baby is given to her lap. The bride leaves the baby in her arms for a while and then leaves it to her own bed. This baby sits first on the newly married couple's bed. Thus, the new bride is believed to be fertile[218].

In this period, which is seen in the early stages of pregnancy, care is taken to give the pregnant woman whatever she wants, no matter how irrelevant she is.

If this rule is not observed, it is believed that a number of harmful effects may occur in the mother or the child to be born. According to this belief, the need or desire of the craving mother cannot be met can cause effects such as the mother's miscarriage, disability or birth of the baby. There is no different situation in Alevism from other cultures related to craving. There are some points that the pregnant woman should pay attention to during this period. There is a belief that if the mother eats frequently during pregnancy, looking at some people or animals will affect the child's temperament, body structure and facial features. As a requirement of this belief, the pregnant woman is afraid to eat, to look at such people and to encounter such animals, which is possible to leave a trace of a defect in the

216 İbid.,Ergun P. (2011). pp, 281–306.
217 İbid., Yalçın H. (2016). Pp. 79-94.
218 Kılıç S., Altuncu, A. ve Gaspak, A. (2016). Beliefs and practices related to birth in flames living in Anatolian countryside (Haçova Case). *Electronic Turkish Studies*, 11(17), 431–446.

baby [219]. Victims are slaughtered so that the child is born both as a healthy and a good son. In addition, before the mother gives birth easy she is asked to avoid dangerous situations in advance, some places, invested, and the places to visit and pray prayers. Children do not fall to snakes, dogs etc. and should avoid animals[220].

In addition to medical methods, the public practice has found ways of determining gender by themselves since very early periods. The child in the belly of the pregnant boy becomes pregnant and the girl becomes ugly. Pregnant, pregnant with the girl wants to sour; If the boy is pregnant, he wants dessert. If the pregnant woman wears a necklace in her dream, her child is a girl; If the child wears a bracelet " a belief is available. Without knowing the pregnant woman, a knife is placed under a cushion and scissors are placed under a cushion. The pregnant is called to the room. The child will be a boy if he sits on a mat with a knife underneath, and a girl if he sits on a mat with scissors underneath. When the last months of birth are entered, the pregnant woman is carried out abundantly and moved to facilitate birth.

In the Alevi culture, birth is carried out by women who are called midwives, who were believed to have traditional birth techniques in villages. Today, however, births are performed in hospitals in city centers. In addition, the counseling functions of midwives continue. The woman who will give birth, to facilitate birth during the birth "Hand is not my hand, Fatma mother's hand" will give birth to the woman's belly rubs the hand. It is believed that birth will be easy with this application [221]. In addition, a handful of ashes are taken from the grandfather's quarry, which is accepted as the leader of religious beliefs, for the ease of birth, Dede poures this ash into a glass of water, mixed with the prayers he reads, and this mixture is made when the woman's pain increases. In addition, a handful of ashes are

---

219 Büyükokutan A. (2005). *Muğla region A research on folk literature and folk-lore products of Alevi Turkmens.* Master Thesis.Balıkesir University Institute of Social Sciences Department of Turkish Language and Literature. 327–417

220 Yıldırım E. (2010). A sociological study on the beliefs and practices of the transition period in the Tunceli region. *EKEV Academy Journal. 14*(42), 17–32.

221 Selçuk A. (2004). A phenomenological approach to the beliefs and practices of planners about birth. *Turkology Researches, 16*(16), 163–178.

taken from the grandfather's quarry, which is considered to be the leader of religious beliefs, for easy birth. Grandfather poured this ash into a glass of water, mixed with the prayers he read and this mixture is made when the woman's pain increases during childbirth. With another application, water is poured into the skirt of a woman who had a baby with a comfortable and comfortable birth before, and this skirt is squeezed and the water in it is put into a glass and given to pregnant woman. In this way, birth is believed to be as comfortable as the other woman. In addition, the buttons of the clothes in the house are removed from the loop and the doors and windows in the house are opened. People at home during childbirth do not bind their hands together. In this way, it is believed that delivery will take place comfortably [222]

After the pregnancy, with the birth of a new concern for the baby and mother begins. Alevi Turkmen are sacrificed after birth. His family is prayed to be a blessed son[223],[224] . The woman who gave birth is called "forty woman". Forty women with baby after forty days after child is born is not removed from bed. Forty women are not allowed to do business. His relatives come to him and do his work. Whether the child is a girl or a boy, the victim is slaughtered in his name, and the baby and his mother survive forty days and then they are made and distributed. This was done for the baby and his mother to survive forty days and survive.

Forty women and children in the fortress of the woman, forty woman in the head tied red, the child is covered with a red cover. Forty days, fire, flour and salt are not given out of the house. The laundry of the forties and the baby is not laid outside the house. If a red writing is not tied to the head of a forty woman, her child is weak and diseased. The red veil covered on the child and the red writing attached to the head of the forty woman are washed after their forty and are not used again. This red cover and writing is given to someone outside the family[225]. The mouth of the maternity remains open for forty days. Forty women and their children, forty days to

222 İbid.,Yıldırım E. (2010).p. 19
223 İbid.,Yıldırım E. (2010).pp. 17–32.
224 İbid.,Selçuk A. (2004). pp.163–178.
225 Yazlak Y.(2011). Haçova village culture and history, Malatya Haçova Village Culture and Solidarity Association,1. 3–5.

keep out of the house. Forty women don't go to a wedding or funeral home in forty days. Newly born women are not left alone. He's laid in his bed. Red duvets are covered. Mother and baby are expected. If they're alone, "take it," and evil spirits will come [226].

When we look at ways of eliminating childlessness, medical treatment methods are used especially for Alevi Turkmen living in district centers. However, if you have not worked for many years and the results are not going to the shrines, medicines made from various herbs are used, and a small amount of treatment with "Musca" is applied. However, if they do not have children, they receive a child from their close relatives. If relatives do not want to give any of their children, they may be asked to do a child for themselves [227].

Following the birth of the child, the cutting process of the belly which provides the connection between mother and child is followed. Belly cutting and the places where the cut belly is placed in many beliefs and practices in our culture. In the Alevi culture, the placenta is called a "partner" and they believe that there is a connection between it and the child. Therefore, the baby's wife, buried in a place where the feet will not touch. The cutting of the hub is also not performed on a random one. Because it is believed that there will be a similarity between the child who cuts the belly and the character of the child in later life. For this reason, although not going to the hospital, people who are loved and considered in the community, knowledgeable people are preferred. This person may also have certain rights to that child when necessary.

The child's belly is buried in a place where people cannot set foot. These places are the places where the child is expected to be in the future. School gardens are the most preferred among these places. Alevism attach great importance to education. It often emphasizes that every child should receive good education without distinction between boys and girls[228,229]

Salting: 8-10 after birth. Salting method is another application made in order to make the child healthy. Among the reasons for salting, the child

---

226 İbid., Kılıç S., Altuncu, A. ve Gaspak, A. (2016). Pp.431-446
227 İbid.,Yalçın H. (2016). Pp.79-94.
228 İbid.,Yıldırım E. (2010).pp. 17–32.
229 İbid.,Selçuk A. (2004). pp.163–178.

does not smell, perspiration, the body is not the body and arrogance is asked to be arrogant. Wait for one or two hours and wash[230] . In Alevi culture, attention is paid to the names given to the child to be beautiful and to be the names of respectable people. Because the name given to the child is believed to affect the future of his life. We know that the grandfather did the name-making process earlier, but nowadays, the grandfather's name is given to his grandfather or father because they are less frequent to the settlements. Usually, the child is given the names commonly used in the community (Ali, Hüseyin, Hasan, Mustafa, Fatma, Ayşe, Elif), grandmother and grandfather. In addition to this, the names of the parents are chosen as the more modern ones. In addition, in order to have children, if the places such as tombs are visited, the names of the persons mentioned in the tomb are given. The Alevi Turkmens also sacrifice when naming them. Women who do not have children go to visit the tomb and hermit grave for their children to live[231]. Traditional beliefs about child care continue in Alevism. Traditional applications for common health problems are as follows:

Colds: The trophy is drawn to the back of the body. Cotton sweeps around the end of a bar. The ones on the patient are removed. When the back is naked, cotton, immersed in alcohol, is ignited. The flamed rod is inserted into the glass cup and removed from the patient's back. Cups, vacuum back. It is done in the same way than a few bars. Mint is boiled, lemon is squeezed into it. Rheumatism: The leeches collected from the reeds in small water bottles are adhered to the body's aching places. The leech sucks blood filthy. When the blood is cleared, the leech swells up and stops sucking and dies. Bee and Insect Bites: In the case of bee and insect bites, the most important flower of this region is the water of the oleander flower. Malaria: To heal, the patient is incinerated with onion and garlic. Wart: The leaf of the fig tree is plucked from the bottom. The milk is drained. Flowing fig milk is applied on the wart. After two or three

230 İbid.,Yıldırım E. (2010).pp. 22.
231 Örnek S.V.(2000). *Turkish Folklore, Ankara: Ministry of Culture Publications.* 162–163.

weeks, all the warts disappear. Three Ihlas while driving, a Fatiha surah is read. *Gas Pains*: Oil of apple oil or almond, thyme oil is smeared on the stomach[232,233].

Headache: Raw onions and potatoes on the forehead of the headaches are connected to the forehead of the patient with a cloth. The check is drawn by writing. *Boil*: The onion is cooked in the embers. Hot wrapped on top of unopened boil. Enables the opening of the product. *Tonsil*: Almonds are wrapped in warm water in the throat of the swollen. One day is waited. The throat of the patient is connected with a towel. The tonsils are detonated by pulling towards the back. *Abdominal Pain*: Children who have pain in the abdomen, mush is made. Poulters on his belly. Hayit beats his leaf and wraps his abdomen. For those who have diarrhea, the wild pear is boiled and fed. Quince leaves boiled, water is drunk. Stomach aches, anise seeds eaten boiled, good for stomach pains. Chamomile tea is good for stomach pains. Style; To pass through the arpace, the water is driven. Honey, butter or yogurt is applied to the burning place[234].

Urinary Tract Disorder: Urinary tract infiltrators are seated in hot water. In addition, if there is water with the spring leaf. When in adulthood, the patient is seated naked in water. The brick is heated in a fire and wrapped in a towel. The patient is seated on top. Red jaundice, red cloth, cranberry syrup. Food is very sweet. It is laid under the light. The connection between the upper teeth and the lip is cut very little by razor blade. Blood flows. So jaundice flows. *Diabet*: Diabetic patients drink blackberry juice and mulberry juice. *Constipation*: Soap is refined by carving. He comes in through the bum of the kid. Dried figs are boiled and crushed. It is fed with water. It removes constipation. The blood of the new born woman is dripped to those whose eyes are bloody and their ear hurts. The ear and eye are treated for a while. Those with high blood pressure will boil forty olive leaves in one

232 Karaağaç G. and Alacain Ş. (2004). *Our house in Ortaca, Muğla*: Anıl Ofset-Tipo Typography. 362.
233 Şöhret D.Ü. (2004). *Folk medicine in Fethiye and the beliefs about it*, Book of Muğla. Prepared by: Ali Abbas Cinar, Izmir: Printer Offset Printing. 297.
234 İbid., Selçuk A. (2004). 163-178.

liter of water. In the morning, drink a glass of water on an empty stomach. Those with low blood pressure drink plenty of salty buttermilk[235,236,237].

According to Alevi circles in our country, death, especially in rural areas, has an important place in the life of society. Therefore, everyone expects death, fear and respect. Rituals related to death It is seen that in the Alevi's living in our country, some rituals are applied at the time of death and after death. There may be some differences in the localities and the region of these practices. These rituals related to death can be examined in two parts, basically in the form of preparation and embedding phase. From the moment the death began to occur, the process of the funeral prayer was done until the "preparatory stage"; The process of burial after the funeral prayer and the burial of the dead can be considered as the "recessed stage". Alevi funerals exhibit a full Anatolian diversity, which is widespread, shrouded, the type of washing the corpse is similar to the Sunni, the slaughter at funerals is still an important ritual. The most important thing in worship is the Turkish language. The burial process in the flame culture is absolutely not done at night. Because according to the flame belief, the earth and the sky are sealed when the night collapses. Therefore, digging and rowing do not work. If someone dies at night, all the operations are done in the daytime, washing, shroud etc. The funeral prayer is overridden by the Alevi's in the homes of Cem. Then they'll take the dead out of the coffin and bury them in the cemetery. After the funeral, he accepts guests for three days at the condolence house, after the third day after eating Yasin recited meal. 40 days after the funeral in flames, 40 is given the bite. Later, at the end of a year, you are given a meal with Yasin recited.

There is no significant difference between the Anatolian Alevism and the Turkish community structure in general. At the beginning of the differences that are the most evident are the different religious tendency (only in some small applications) and the lifestyle comes. However, this difference is limited, and it can be expressed that the social structure and norms are more effective on the determinants of the life style. Health-related features, health-conscious levels and perspectives on healthcare workers are still

---

235 İbid.,Yıldırım E. (2010). pp.17-32.
236 Selçuk A. (2004). pp.163-178.
237 Yıldız H. (2007).pp, 93-112.

parallel to the general characteristics of Turkish society and are important. It is determined that there are positive attitudes towards health care workers in particular. Although the methods such as the healer, the wish and the Amulet are not approved, it is possible to apply these methods for women who do not have children, and these methods can be gained in places where modern medicine remains inadequate. Consequently, the Alevi Turkmens, who are curious because they have a semi-closed society that reacts because they are different, are actually present in Turkish culture; However, they continue to have some forgotten beliefs and practices today.

3 Research Example

3.1 Evaluation of Anatolian Alevi People Living in Istanbul with "Purnell' Cultural Competence Model"

The purpose of this study is to evaluate Anatolian Alevi people living in Istanbul with Cultural "Purnell' Cultural Competence Model". Sample of this qualitative conducted study includes total of 30 Alevi people aging between 19 and 56, registered at Ümraniye Ihlamurkuyu Cem houses. Snowball sampling method was used to select the sample. The research data were collected in the form of a semi-structured interview form, written recordings and voice recordings, which included the topics included in Purnell's cultural competence model to assess cultural features.

Focus group interviews were conducted between January and March 2017. Data were collected by using voice and written records. Collected data were analyzed by using descriptive analysis and semiotics methods. It is reported that early marriage, marriage with relatives and early pregnancy are common, and alcohol and smoking are rare in Alevi population. In addition, it was also reported that there are some negative perceiving such as double standard in society, low health service opportunity, and religious discrimination. Results found in the research showed that there are not significant differences between Anatolian Alevi and Turkish population on social demographic and social structures. In order to decrease this perceiving, more social and cultural combining programs may be conducted.

3.1.1 Materials and Methods

Type of research: This research was carried out with qualitative research methods focus group interview method.

3.1.2 The Universe and Sample of Research

The universe of this research, which is a qualitative type, has been composed of 30 Turkish citizens of 15 years of age and over who are registered in Istanbul Ümraniye Ihlamurkuyu Cem House. The sampling of the population was carried out with the maximum diversity sampling method of snowballs to provide the maximum diversity with a small sample by the sampling method. The study group included 30 Turks of Alevi origin with different demographic characteristics between the ages of 15–65. The subjects of Turkish origin, Alevi, volunteer participation and cognitive competence were searched.

3.1.3 Data collecting

The data were collected by focus group interview method between April/ May 2017 with the semi-structured interview form which was formed by the researchers in line with "Purnell' Cultural Competence Model". Also information and consent form used. The contents of the interview form consisted of 12 areas of "Purnell' Cultural Competence Model"[238]. Each of these 12 areas created a theme and the theme contents of the 12 areas of the model were determined using the work done on Romans (Gypsies) by Tanriverdi and his friends[239].

i.   General information, region of residence: the migration to the region, reasons, educational status, evaluated the professional situation.

ii. Communication: main language, dialect, tone of voice was evaluated here.

iii. Family roles and organizations: head of the family, gender roles, children and lifestyles were evaluated here.

iv. Workforce Status: job finding status and employment status were assessed here.

v.   Biocultural Ecology: biological properties, disease and health conditions were assessed here.

vi. High risk behaviors: smoking and alcohol use, drug addiction, sexual practices were assessed here.

vii. Nutrition: food rituals, nutritional habits were assessed here.

viii. Pregnancy and birth practices: pregnancy, traditional practices, applications for the end of birth and childbirth were evaluated.

---

238 Purnell L.(2008) Transcultural diversty and health care. In: Purnell L, Paulkanca BJ, eds. *Transcultural Health Care: A Culturally Competent Approach*. 3 rd ed. Philadelphia: F.A. Davis Company; p. 19–55.
239 İbid., Tanrıverdi et al.,(2012).pp.243-253

ix. Death rituals: death rituals and death assessment were discussed here.

x. Spirituality: spiritual beliefs and healthcare practices were discussed here.

xi. Health care Practices: health and disease, cultural responses, organ donation and organ transplantation, such topics were evaluated here.

xii. Health care workers: the condition of healthcare providers, the approach to sorcerers and sorcery were discussed here.

In order to determine the individuals to be interviewed, the purpose and importance of working under the responsible grandfather of Istanbul Ihlamurkuyu Cem House was explained. We have preliminary information on the neighborhood. Cem House grandparents made suggestions on when and where to do the interviews. Before the interviews were made, the "Information and consent form" was taken to the participants who agreed to participate in the research and received approval signatures. Thursday is an important day for the Alevis and they perform their religious meetings on Thursday. A total of 14 men and 16 women were interviewed on Thursday for two consecutive weeks in the neighborhood and the cemevi. Interviews "Ihlamurkuyu Cem House " was made in the form of 5–10-person groups in the grandfather room. The groups were determined to be able to talk together comfortably. Each of the negotiations took approximately 60–90 minutes. The interviews were terminated after both participants and researchers continued until there was no new information. Data were gathered by researchers in the form of voice recorder and note-taking. Prior to the study, a written permission was obtained from the Ethics committee of the University where one of the researchers was affiliated and the individuals included in the study. Talks; The code was given to participants based on confidentiality. The information collected by the participants of the "demographic characteristics form", which includes demographic characteristics such as gender, age, marital status, and questions to be given to the privacy-based participant.

3.1.4 Data Evaluation

The data was evaluated by descriptive analysis method. The audio recordings and written notes collected by the researchers were transferred to the computer environment. All recordings were made according to the themes in Purnell's model. The statements of the persons were evaluated and summarized in general. Speech texts were shown in italics. Female and male participants were encoded and numbered.

3.1.5 Results and Discussion

Among the Alevi's included in the study group, 14 of them were male, 16 were female, aged between 19 and 56, married and have children. It was found that most of the people in the group had a regular income and that they retired, two people were university students and 10 others were high school graduates and others were primary school graduates.

3.1.5.1 General Information, Region of Residence: Reasons for the presence of migration to the region of residence, educational status, professional status assessed.

Settlement, Migration, Causes of Migration

(F1) Our roots are from various cities of Anatolia. We have been living in Istanbul for over 40 years. Our origins did not come from Tunceli in Sivas. During Dersim events our grandmothers migrated from Adiyaman to Erzincan from Tunceli. We migrated to Istanbul with the mentality of where is not your's born, is where you live your life (M1) We are Turkish roots and We are the first to accept Islam. We are Alevi, God, Muhammad, Ali was born with the belief, we live and we die. We are Ehlibeyt descendants. Our ancestors lived in the Anatolian lands, but they always hid themselves and our faith in fear of oppression and death. Our ancestors migrated to Istanbul and we have lived for 30 years, we have cem hause for 20 years and we can make our prayers easily. (M2) My origins come from Iran Khorasan. I'm Turkmen. We come from the origins of Seyit-Mahmut Hayrani. Alevi is human. We were birthed in Sivas, but we were a crowded family. We migrated to Istanbul for a life fight. We've been living in this area for 30 years. Neither our language nor our religion is different. We agreed to Islam and the Islamic community. (M3) All the Alevi's in this neighborhood that we live in have migrated from different cities of Turkey. At first, everyone was hiding themselves. The people at the government offices didn't say they were Alevi. But when we see each other in the trenches, we learn that they are Alevi. We're seeing each other in the neighborhood. We're also seeing our Sunni brothers. Our origins are Turks, Muslims. We do not distinguish Sunni, Alevi. But the Sunnies are making a distinction for us. (M1) Me and my family everywhere say that we are Alevi Turks. No harm from us. Our tribe is human, we do not harm human beings, we fear Allah. We migrated from our village because of unemployment. (F2) My ancestors immigrated to Istanbul 46 years ago with the cause of unemployment and poverty. I am born in Istanbul and I live in Ümraniye. I grew up in this neighborhood. Our origins are Turkmen and Alevi conquest and my ancestry are Turkic descendants. Our essence is Turkish. I do not explain that we have the Alevi faith as long as I do not have to. Even the most contemporary people behave differently when they hear this. But we are the real Muslim. We believe in the Ehlibeyt, Allah Muhammad and Ali, obey. In prayer, we pray that our nation will not cause harm to our nation. Our ancestors escaped to the mountainous regions during Ottoman times. Our villages are always in the mountainous region.

As can be seen from the prominent statements, a large proportion of the Alevi's and their circles living in Istanbul came from geographies such as Uzbekistan, Iran, Turkmenistan and Khorasan. When asked about the phenomenon of immigration, it is seen that the responses are generally based on religious elements. The second highlight is the theme of unemployment. Unemployment is one of the most important causes of internal and external migration. Unemployment, which is examined under the name of economic reasons, affects a large part of humanity regardless of factors such as religion, language, race, age and gender[240]. There are varieties such as seasonal or seasonal migrations and agricultural migrations. Thus the unemployment of the reasons for the migration of Alevism is not only a cause of the Alevis, for all individuals with low or moderate income in Turkey is valid reasons. On the other hand, migrations based on religious factors, the developments after the events such as Dersim and Maraş, have investigated the flames as an important cause of migration for the citizens.

---

240 Turkish Statistical Institute(TÜİK), (2017). Employment and Household data.
    http://www.tuik.gov.tr/PreTablo.do?alt_id=1007(Date of access 17.12.2018)

Education

(**M4**) My education is primary school, but we attach great importance to the education and training of our children. Our only weapon is to read and have a profession. There is no uncle in the state's top offices, our children are working in lower positions. Not brought to the top authority. But they can't take the diploma. (**F3**) We are hiding in schools that our children have a flame when they learn that they are excluded by their friends. Their education, especially religious education should be done according to the belief of Alevism. (**F5**) We care a lot about education. We are studying the children of Alevis in the region and do not have a university graduate, so illiterate. Few of our elderly people who are 70 or older in our family do not know how to read and write, but they know how to read. (**M5**) Our new generation of youth and children are studying. Women are working and boys are working. I'm a primary school graduate, even if we have the raw material. There are many who read in our neighborhood and we are in this majority. In the cem house in our grandfather, is education and says to us for education. There is no gossip in our conversations. (**M6**) At least primary school is the most high school graduate. I couldn't read it, but let my child read. I'm working on the construction sites.

When the answers to the question related to education are examined, Alevi's stated that they attach great importance to education, but they cannot see enough of the education they received because they are Alevi. Although the research sample is between 19 and 56 years of age by age average, there are more than 30 participants. Therefore, the average age of education according to the average age of high school shows that the level of education is higher than the age groups. In the responses to the question related to education, it is seen that the emphasis on Alevi identity is at the forefront. In fact, the unemployment rate is constantly increasing with the increase of population in Turkey, and by level of education increased education level of the unemployed population is also increasing. For this reason, the number of unemployed people with diplomas increases day by day[241](158). Therefore, it can be stated that there is at least not a statistical

241 İbid., Turkish Statistical Institute(TÜİK), (2017).

meaning of an application for Alevi citizens. However, the fact that this perception is a genius indicates negative practices in the past.

Job

(E6) I'm a builder, I don't have a permanent job. Most of the men in the Alevi sitting here worked in the construction and still work. Constructions are dangerous. One of our relatives fell out of construction and was paralyzed, in need of help. (F6) I've read it till school. My wife is working as a worker. I wanted so much to read, they will be very sorry afterwards. Now I want to go to school to have a profession. (M7) I finished high school, but I couldn't continue my education because my parents were leaving. Now I work in a private institution. But I want to continue training. I don't want to work as an unskilled employee. I got through this familiar job, it's hard to find a job when it's not familiar. When they learn about our identity, they treat us differently, looking at us differently. (M8) I retired by working on the constructions, and now I'm out of work. Unemployment. I couldn't read a job. Civil engineering. There was lack of immigration from the village. We worked on the construction, and we made a living. There was no showing us the way. I worked in very difficult conditions and read my children. But they can't find a good job; because it is very difficult to find work without familiar. (F10) I want to work on a monthly job. I want to get money in time of unemployment and to retire and be insured. I don't want to look at my husband's hand. I don't have a profession. (F12) I studied English language teaching. My family's work place is available sometimes I go there to help them. I want to continue my education.

When the answers to the occupational question are examined, it is seen that construction, self-employed or unqualified workers are in majority. According to the educational status of Alevi citizens, their professional distribution is close to each other. Individuals who are generally educated at primary and high school level are individuals who are employed in blue collar or unskilled jobs. The white collar or the individuals working in the professions such as engineers, architects and doctors are more educated. In this respect, socio-demographic samples and their observations from their environment indicate that the professions addressing the middle and low socio-economic classes are in the majority.

3.1.5.2 Communication

The participants expressed that they learned Turkish from Alevi's, and they learned from the Kurds in the region where they lived together. In fact, most of the participants stated that they could understand Kurdish but could not speak. When communicating, sex is not important, there is no distinction between men and women. But in times of sadness, we prefer to remain silent. While expressing love, they stated that there was no obstacle to eye contact or touch. Although they stated that there was no gender difference in general among the health personnel, they stated that they want this preference to be in their gender. (F14) In general, we speak Turkish, Turkish is our native language. The volume of our speeches is high, there is praise and greeting while showing our love. (F7) We do not discriminate on health issues. It doesn't matter if you're a man or a woman.

It is seen that communication subject is formed under two headings and responded accordingly. The first one is different and communication with other societies, and the second is communication within the society. In inter-communal communication, it is seen that they use Turkish language effectively and they know Kurdish language in comprehension level. In this respect, it can be stated that Alevi's have no difficulty in communicating with different societies. In social communication among themselves, answers are emphasized in the patriarchal structure which is valid in the large part of Turkish society, especially in Alevi society. It has been underlined that gender is not a factor for blocking communication among individuals.

3.1.5.3 Family Roles and Organizations

At home, who was in charge of the head of duty, the role and task distribution according to gender was evaluated.

Head of the Family

(F15) The head of the family is usually male. Although the head of the family is a man, the woman has a say more. Men used to be interested in anything related to the house just goes to work and earn money. Now he can help his wife, if necessary, take care of the children. Sends children to school for education. (M9) Woman weighs more at home. My wife's requests are very important. In the past, marriages would be early. We grew up with my wife.

But now we're teaching our kids. No early marriage. Elderly is our crown. If you are the only son, the parents will stay with you. We have to take care of them. (F10) The head of the house is a man. We don't employ old people. They are cared for, more attention is paid. Children are raised, educated and occupied. Help the elderly in difficult situations. In the distribution of the head of the family and the roles in the household, it is seen that there is a structure similar to the patriarchal Turkish family structure, but this structure seems to be patriarchal in nature, but in essence, gender equality is more experienced. It is seen that the family structure is suitable for the traditional Turkish large family structure, the mother and father stay with the youngest child, after a while the family head produces or produces bread at home. The nuclear family is not as dominant as the Turkish community.

Marriage

(M11) Marriages usually happen between the flames. Other than this, marriage is excluded, not required. In the marriage, the official marriage is done in a religious but religious ceremony. (F15) His consolation was 10–20 years ago. It's done very little now. There is a marriage among Alevi's but they are not related. His wife, deceased ladies usually do not marry. They will not marry him. (F16) I got married at 14. I had my first child when I was 15. I married very early and my wife is a relative. But thankfully, none of our children had any health problems. (F14) We are not given a foreign girl. Strangers are not welcome. Girls who are already foreigners have problems in their marriages. That's what I tell my children. I am against Sunni Alevi marriages. But if they love each other, we won't.

In terms of marriage, in the regions with low socio-demographic characteristics of Anatolia, where education level is low, negativities such as early marriage and consanguineous marriage are common. Although Alevi individuals paid more attention to gender equality in terms of communication and social roles within the family, the belief and patriarchal structure outweigh the marriage and the establishment of the family. One of the most remarkable points here is that marriage of consanguineous marriage, which is strictly prohibited in medicine, constitutes serious risks for both parents and children, is considered more normal than marrying different beliefs, which are just a belief and a view. While a person is free to marry a relative, it is not welcome to marry another person of faith. Again, the marriage of widows is considered negative, while the same situation does not apply to men whose wife has died.

Severity

(M12) We say no to violence against women. Me and my people do not like to raise hands and despise women. (F16) Violence against women is not welcome and there is almost none. In our neighborhood there is a family with flame like us. His wife has been unemployed for 6 months. The woman heard that she was upset by her partner, but she rarely goes down like that. Lack of life makes people like this. (F13) There is no violence. I help the woman who's seen violence. Man is at the top of our philosophy and there is no more valuable asset than it. No one deserves beatings of violence.

All the participants against violence, because they keep people at the highest level, negative views. Another prominent point here is that women's violence is perceived and questioned when asked about violence. On the other hand, despite the widespread violence against women in Turkish society, in the interviews or interviews, a large part of the population is against the so-called female violence. However, even in the case of consensus that it is against such violence, the marriages between different beliefs are not approved, and therefore, one of the violence of women, which is one of the violence of the family, is given to the violence.

3.1.5.4 Workforce Status

(M11) We work without discrimination of men. My salary is not enough for my children and my wife. He works for my wife. We're both primary school graduates. We want to retire and work as an insured. We don't want to look at anyone's hands. (F10) In my youth, my wife didn't let me work. I worked after 40. I raised my children. I'm retired now. My salary is less, but we are not in need of anybody. Our children are hard to find a job, there is unemployment. Even if they are ill, they do not work for the unfamiliar or they work with very low salary.

In terms of labor force, there is no significant difference between the Alevi community and Turkish society in general. In general, the social structure in Turkey, which has an average and under income, is the most important goal for retiring and maintaining their lives without looking at anyone's hands. Again, in Alevism, the intense gender inequality structure of the patriarchal structure is manifested as the necessity of being familiar and close to the work, the need for no one and the work of the woman depends on the permission of the spouse.

3.1.5.5 Biological Features

Skin Color

(F1) There is a general saying that the skin color of our skin color is slightly dark. But me and my family are general clear skinned. (F4) As we are Turkish Alevism, we are light-skinned but we are black-eyed. Even the eyes of most of my family are light blue and green. (M5) There is no brunette in our family. They even compare us to the Thracians.

While there is no distinct class of property as a result of skin color, it is stated that Turkish Alevi's are light-skinned but generally Alevi's are dark and green eyes. On the other hand, though in this case the right to Alevi's in general, Alevism in Turkey is meant to be valid. When the answers to the question of migration about where the Alevi's come from, Iran and Turkic republics come to the fore. In these regions, people have a relatively dark, green-eyed structure. Generally, this may be the reason why Alevi's have dark and green eyes. On the other hand, Alevi's living in Turkey for many years, phenotype and genotype were also reflected the view shaped by environment.

Disease and Health Conditions

(F3) Our family has a predisposition to stomach cancer and diabetes. It is not because we are Alevi. In general, an obvious disease is not seen in our ethnic origin. Diseases related to the conditions in which we live like in other people.

When the answers given to the question were examined, it was stated that there is no type of disease that is specific to Alevi's or Alevi individuals. In fact, there are studies reporting that some diseases are more common in some societies due to the region and genetic structure. Nowadays, DSÖ reports results according to races in their reports. However, there is no specific discomfort in the literature for the flame community. Participants also stated that they did not observe a disease in this way.

3.1.5.6 High Risk Behaviors

(**F1**) Smoking and alcohol use among men in our family is not much. There are Alevi teens in the neighborhood and not in my family, but using drugs. They also use alcohol on special occasions. There are those who never use it. Women are not allowed to drink alcohol. (**M9**) I can't use alcohol nor cigarette neither. I will tell you about the harm in my children. Smoking is very harmful to health. (**F4**) We have monogamy in our family. We're against polygamy. Besides, we can't give birth to a child we can't look for. My family plans.

When the answers were examined, it was stated that smoking and alcohol use among the Alevi's were not common and became increasingly common among young people. Substance addiction was also very low. Monogamy is common among the flames, and they are against polygamy. Family planning is considered important among the flames. No physical activity, high-risk behavior will constitute the activity is not specified. Early age and consanguineous marriage, which were high risk for the future of the child, were considered normal.

3.1.5.7 Nutrition

(**F2**) Pig, dog, hedgehog, cat, rabbit inedible. We pay attention to balanced nutrition and nutrition according to our economic situation. (**F12**) As the price is suitable for vegetables we find more natural if we find. We can eat anything less. (**M1**) We love to share. We share our food with our neighbors and the poor. We do not forget to feed the animals they carry. (**M3**) The concepts of tableware, cooking and cooking were sanctified between Alevi's as well as in all Anatolian cultures and took place in every stage of our life. The Bektashi table is established and all the people participate. Men and women sit at the table together.

Nutritional habits in general had the same characteristics as Turkish society. It was stated that rabbit meat was not eaten as in some parts of Anatolia. Nutrition is a condition that is directly related to the economic situation or income. In this respect, the flames expressed that they ate less than anything else as long as economic conditions allowed. It is also the mystical meaning of the table, animals and other living things are the most basic rights of feeding is the answer to the cultural elements of nutrition.

Generally, due to the low economic level, it was stated that there was a below-average diet.

3.1.5.8 Pregnancy and Birth Practices

(F16) The woman who does not get pregnant goes to the doctor first and then goes to the places we call spirituality. This is very important for the continuation of our generation. We believe that when you go to this visit and pray, it will be accepted. Make a wish, sacrifice. Pregnant women do not work hard (M13) If the pregnant woman sees a meal, she is taken. The pregnant woman is not left alone. A woman without a child goes to a visit and prays and the child is named after the visit, and the victim is slaughtered. (F11) Woman who gave birth are not left alone. The Quran is read. Light is lit to protect from evil spirits. The child's belly is not thrown out of thought. It's buried in the ground. It's part of the human. 40 is removed when the child is 40. Mother and child bathe. 40 wheats are put in water and washed with water. (F6) Women in the village next to the woman who stayed with them for 3 days. In the past, the children were set on fire and salted. Now this is not done. The duvet and the bed become red and dressed in red, and the red scarf is attached to her. Woman who gave birth is fed with blood-forming foods. Milk-making foods are given. 3 days after the prayer is called by saying the name is taken from her mother and put into her own bed.

It was seen that there were some belief rituals for the child to have a wish about being pregnant, sacrifice, visiting the tomb. Pregnancy and childbirth are important for the continuation of the generation and are part of the social and social structure. Taking pregnant women to eat the food they see, not working hard, burning light to protect from evil spirits are the elements which belong to Turkish society life rather than belief. They were also seen in Alevism. It was stated that the woman who gave birth would be dressed in red and that the bed would be red, and that the child would be pushed to prevent it.

3.1.5.9 Death Rituals

(M10) In a house, death is mourned. No entertainment, no radio, no music, no music. This continues for 40 days. On the 3rd day of death, no food is served and meals are served. For 40 days, one's belly is made by eating from the house of the dead. On the 7th and 52nd days the Qur'an is distributed and the halva is distributed. The clothes of the dead are distributed. (M12) We wash our dead in cem houses and perform their prayers. We have post-mortem food here.

Widespread Turkish society rituals of the death of the funeral in the mosque or sanctuary, burial operations, the deceased of the clothes, 7'si, 40'si meals and beliefs are. Halva is a food distributed after death in the Turkish community. In the Alevi community, many rituals other than the mosque being washed and prayed at the cem house instead of the mosque are in harmony with the Turkish society. The Alevism in the sample stated that days 3, 7, 40 and 52 are important after the death. Similar to the practices of the Turkish community in Anatolia, mourning in the dead house, radio, TV and music were not opened.

3.1.5.10 Spirit

(M13) Spirituality is to give value to human beings. We carry out our religious duties. But if you do these things and you are in all kinds of evil, there is no value. We also love people who are strong in spirituality. We seek refuge in Allah, but not always. (F5) My spiritual orientation is strong. I pray a lot to God. I need help from him.

Alevism stated that their spirituality, especially religious feelings, was important and that they were determinative in their lives. As well as car-rying out religious duties, it is important for them to avoid evil. In fact, all belief systems have this approach in theory. Because religion and spir-ituality aims to remove people from wrong and correct. In their response to marriage and family, Alevi's said that they did not welcome marriage from other faiths, and that spirituality was also a determinant of life and social structure.

3.1.5.11 Health Care Practices

(M14) Health is when a person feels happy. In order to be healthy, we consume foods with high vitamin value. I also ensure that my children eat naturally. (F14) If I can do my daily work, I'm fine. I lost most of my relatives from cancer. That's why we need to appreciate life. Our economic situation is not good. I take care of our health. When we get sick, we go to the hospital and the doctor. In the past, it was difficult to go to the hospital and to the doctor. There was no transportation, the hospitals were very queue. Now it's hard to make an appointment. But we have to go. He understands the value of health better when people lose. (F19) Health is very important. Sometimes we use special foods to protect our health. In times of illness, we only go to the doctor. We don't go to the healer, the broken bitch. Conditions such as printing amulets are not preferred. We only pray only in disease cases. (F11) If I don't have stress or sadness, my health is good. When one of my family is ill, Then I will accept whatever comes to God. (F16) The basis of health includes hygiene and cleanliness. I go to the doctor right after you get sick. But I use herbs that I know are good or that they support medical treatment. I believe in the eyes. Sometimes I go to your grandparents and pray for my children. The evil eye can crack a person. (F8) When I'm cold, when I'm fired, I take a warm bath and drink hot drinks. I do it to my kids. The body is wiped with vinegar water over high heat.

In healthcare practices, no statement specific to the Alevi community was found. In general, individuals with moderate- or lower-income levels are determined by health and vitamins, stress and sadness, hygiene and cleanliness. Similar answers were given in Alevism. They stated that in the case of simple colds or fever, some measures were taken at home, hospitals were experiencing general problems (formerly, not being able to make appointments), and they did not give much importance to alternatives other than modern medicine. However, none of the participants mentioned basic supportive issues such as sports and physical activity in health and care practices.

3.1.5.12 Health Care Workers

(F1) I believe evil eye. But we don't believe in magic and sorcerers. We are only praying to our grandfather's cem house so that he can be spiritual well. But we may have a flame in our environment and believe in magic. I do not believe. (M3) For us, doctor, nurse is very important. We entrust our lives to them. May Allah not let them down our heads. We believe in medicine and doctors. We don't have a job with a healer, the wizard. But in our society, there are those who believe in magic and those who do not. (F15) My mother-in-law took me to visit in his village because he didn't have any children when I got married. After my child was born, we went to visit again and cut the victim.

Health workers, nurses and doctors, especially in all societies are seen as important and valuable professional workers. Healthcare workers are seen not only as giving healing to the diseases but also as people whom they entrust their lives to. This situation was similar in Alevi participants. Participants stated that health workers were very important for them, entrusted their lives to them and did not value superstitious beliefs as an alternative to medicine.

3.1.5.13 Conclusion and Suggestions

In this study, Purnell's Cultural Qualification Model of the Anatolian Alevism living in Istanbul evaluated it. According to the results of the study, it was determined that the Anatolian Alevism migrated from the regions where the Alevism, such as Turkmenistan, Uzbekistan, Iran and Khorasan, are living today. The reasons for the immigration of migrants were the unemployment and economic reasons, and the pressures on belief were particularly influential on internal migration. The patriarchal structure in the Alevism and in the roles and organizations within the family was weaker than the general structure of Turkish society. According to Alevism, whether it is a man or a woman, human beings should be valued as human beings and every creature is equal.

On the other hand, this weak structure leaves its place to a strong patriarchal structure in terms of marriage, nesting or early marriage. Similarly, consanguineous marriage is very common among Alevism and decreases as a result of increasing awareness. Again, within the framework of religious beliefs, Anatolian Alevism do not take a warm approach to marriage from other beliefs, but do not take a stern attitude as in the past. In addition, consanguineous marriages or younger marriages are seen as more innocent and applicable than marriages of different beliefs, indicating that there is a serious social problem. In this structure, Anatolian Alevism are similar to the social structure seen in the dominant sociodemographic groups of Turkish society.

Health-related characteristics, awareness of health and their point of view toward health workers are parallel to the general characteristics of Turkish society and are considered important. In particular, positive attitudes toward health workers were determined. Although it is stated that the methods such as humiliation, wish keeping, amulet are not approved, the use of these methods for women without children shows that these methods gained value in places where modern medicine is insufficient.

In general, when the results of the research were evaluated, there was no significant difference between the Anatolian Alevism and the Turkish society. The most significant differences are the different religious trends (only in some minor applications) and lifestyle. However, this difference is limited and it can be stated that social structures and norms are more effective on the determinants of life style.

List of Table

References

1. Şahin, N. H., Bayram, G. O., & Avcı, D. (2009). Culture-sensitive approach: transcultural nursing. Koç University Journal of Education and Research in Nursing (NERJ), 6(1), 2–7.

2. Bolsoy, N., & Sevil, Ü. (2006). Health-disease and culture interaction. Journal of Ataturk University School of Nursing, 9(3), 78–87.

3. Aksoy, Z. (2013). Role of Cultural Intelligence in Multicultural Environments. Unpublished PhD Thesis, Ege University Institute of Social Sciences, Public Relations and Publicity, İzmir.

4. Erdem, N., & Karaca Sivrikaya, S. (2015). Intercultural Approach in the Care of Internal Disease Patients. Turkey Clinics. J Public Health Nurse-Special Topics, 1(3), 14–21.

5. Held, D. (2010). Globalization, sociology: initial readings. (A. Giddens, Ed.) (2nd ed.). İstanbul: Say Publications.

6. Bayık Temel, A. (2008). Multicultural nursing education. Journal of Anatolia Nursing and Health Sciences, 11(2), 92–101.

7. Koçak, Y., & Terzi, E. (2012). Migration in Turkey, effects and solutions of those who migrate to urban. Kafkas University Journal of Economics and Administrative Sciences, 3(3), 163–184

8. Papadopoulos, I., & Lees, S. (2002). Developing culturally competent researchers. Journal of Advanced Nursing, 37(3), 258–264.

9. Jeffreys, M. R. (2000). Development and psychometric evaluation of the transcultural self-efficacy tool: a synthesis of findings. Journal of Transcultural Nursing, 11(2), 127–136.

10 .Öztürk, E., & Öztaş, D. (2012). Transcultural nursing. Batman University Journal of Life Sciences, 1(1), 293–300.

11. Demirkan, E. (2007). Effects of Cultural Differences on Organizational Communication in Multinational Enterprises. Istanbul Yıldız Technical University. dspace.yıldız.edu.tr

12. Williams, R. (2016). Key words: Culture and society vocabulary (6). Istanbul: Sena Ofset.

13. Doğan, Ö. (2012). Cultural sciences and cultural philosophy (6th ed.). Istanbul: Notos Book.

14. Oğuz, E. S. (2011). The Concept of Culture in Social Sciences. Journal of Hacettepe University Faculty of polite letters, 28(2), 123–139.

15. Burke, P. (2006). Cultural history (2). İstanbul: İstanbul Bilgi University Publications.

16. Limon, B. (2012). Concept of popular culture and kitsch in the course of cultural change. Journal of Idil, 1(3), 106–115.

22. Güvenç, B. (2015). The abc of the culture (7th ed.). İstanbul: Yapı Kredi Publications.

23. TDK. (2018). Turkish language institution general Turkish dictionary. https://www.google.com/search?q=t%C3%BCrk+dil+kur umu+s%C3%B6zl%C3%BCk&oq=t%C3%BCrk+dil+kurumu&aqs =chrome.1.69i57j0l4j46.7373j0j8&sourceid=chrome&ie=UTF-8

24. UNESCO. (1982). World Conference on Cultural Policies Final Report. Mexico City. https://unesdoc.unesco.org/ search/N-EXPLORE-b1ce61ef-5cdc-4f6f-b245-25b51fe650ce

25. Göçer, A. (2013). The views of Turkish teacher candidates on language culture: A phenomenological research. Journal of Erzincan University Faculty of Education, 15(2), 25–38.

27. Seviğ, Ü., & Tanrıverdi, G. (2014). Intercultural nursing. İstanbul: Akademi Publishing.

28. Susar, F. A. (2005). Evaluation of cultural barriers encountered in multicultural environments in terms of public relations and advertising; public relations, corporate communication and management in multicultural environments (1st ed.). Istanbul: Istanbul Commerce University Publications.

32. Başalan, F., & Bayık, Temel, A. (2009). Cultural competence in nursing. Journal of Social Policy Studies, 17(17), 51–58.

33. Erci, B. (2014). Public health nursing (2). Amasya: Göktuğ Publishing.

34. Yalçıner, N., & Çam, O. (2015). The views of nurses working in psychiatry on intercultural care. Journal of Ege University Faculty of Nursing, 31(3), 20–36.

26. Çınarlı, İ. (2016). The role of strategic- health communication in the medical health. Journal of Communication Theory and Research 2016(43), 203–216.

37. Karatay, G. (2009). Kars province. identifying the practices of women living in health centers in some health-related emergency situations. Dokuz Eylul University Electronic Journal of School of Nursing, 1(1), 3–16.

40. Aytaç, Ö., & Kurtdaş, M. Ç. (2015). Social origins of health-disease and health sociology. Fırat University Journal of Social Sciences, 25(1), 231–250.

41. Tabak, S. (2002). Health culture and youth. 8th National Public Health Congress. Diyarbakır/Turkey. Akademi Publishing. 23–28.

43. Hotun Şahin, N., Onat Bayram, G., & Avci, D. (2009). Culture-sensitive approach: transcultural nursing. Journal of Education and Research in Nursing, 6(1), 2–7.

44. Demirer, Y. (2006). Conceptualisation of health in the axis of culture and politics: examples of patients and diseases. Society and Physician, 21(1), 25–35.

45. Higginbottom, G. M. (2000). Heart health-associated health beliefs and behaviours of adolescents of African and African Caribbean descent in two cities in the United Kingdom. Journal of Advanced Nursing, 32(5), 1234–1242.

49. Birkök, M. C. (2015). Health sociological paradigms and social factors affecting health. Turkey Clinics J Public Health Nurs-Special Topics, 1(3), 1–6.

50. Hitchcock, J., Schuber, P., & Thomas, S. (2003). Spiritüel and cultural perspectives, USA: Community Health Nursing (Pelmar Pub).

51. Tanrıverdi, G. (2017). Ethnic and cultural assessment and clinical decision making. Eti Aslan, F. (Ed.), Evaluation of health and clinical decision making within. Yenişehir/Ankara: Akademisyen Bookstore. 1–16.

55. Özcan, S. (2013). Pomak identity. First edition, Edirne: Ceren Publishing and Bookstore. 5–89.

56. Yilmaz, A. (2014). International migration: types, causes and effects. Electronic Turkish Studies, 9(2), 1685-1704.

57. Ünal, S. (2012a). Common historical and cultural construction of identity: in Turkey, the Balkans (Rumeli) immigrants. National Folklore, 24(94).

58. Çelik, C. (2003). Immigration identity between institutionalization and congregation. Marife Scientific Accumulation-2. 235–247.

59. Ünal, S., & Demir, G. (2009). Migration, identity and belonging in the context of Balkan immigrants in Turkey. Social transformations and sociological approaches, VI. National Sociological Congress, Andan Menderes University, Aydın, 378–407.

60. Ünal, S. (2012b). The balkan (Rumelia) identity in the city of izmir as a form of social-spatial-political clustering. Contemporary Local Governments, 21(3), 49–77.

61. Özlem, K. (2011). Balkan immigrants and political elections in Turkey. www.tarihistan.org

62. Özdal, B. (2018). An international migration and population movement in the context of Turkey. DORA Printing. Company. Bursa/Turkey. 1st Edition, xii + 368. https://www.academia.edu/37994515/CUMHUR%C4%B0YET_D%C3%96NEM%C4%B0NDE_BALKANLAR_DAN_T%C3%9CRK%C4%B0YE_YE_Y%C3%96NEL%C4%B0K_G%C3%96%C3%87_HAREKETLER%C4%B0

63. Sait, R. (2010). Association and Balkan immigrants in Turkey http://www.gazeteyenigun.com.tr. (Date of access 06.11.2018)

65. Balikci, A. (2007). Visual ethnography among the Balkan Pomak. Visual Anthropology Review, 23(1), 92–96.

66. Memişoğlu, H. (2005). Pomak folk songs in the Balkans. Istanbul: Turkish World Research Foundation.

67. Alp, İ. (2012). The Turks of Pomak (Kumanlar And Kipchaks). Edirne: Trakya University Publications.

68. https://www.turkcebilgi.com/pomaklar (Date of access: 14.11.2018)

69. Öztürk, N., & Aşçıkoca, H. (2013) Environmental, spatial - programmatic and structural evaluation on the houses of Osmaniye town of Pomak. International Journal of Social Research, 6(25), 410–428.

70. Erdinç, D. (2002), The economic situation of the Turkish minority in Bulgaria in the change process, the Turkish encyclopedia. Ankara: Turkey Recent Publications, 20, (394-400)

71. Dürük, E. F. (2007). *The pesne practice in Pomaks: symbolic culture and ethnicity* (Unpublished PhD Thesis). İzmir: Dokuz Eylül University Institute of Fine Arts.

72. http://pomaknews.com/pomashkiselo/?p=1584 (Date of access: 16.11.2018)

73. Eroğlu, M. A. (2015). Balıkesır sındırgı (sahınkaya vıllage) the pomak weavıng. Journal of İdil Art and Language, 4(18), 185–204.

75. Dzhuvalekov, S. (2011). Religious Life of Pomaks (Doctoraldissertation, Selcuk University Institute of Social Sciences).

76. http://pomak.blogspot.com/. (Date of access: 16.11.2018)

77. http://pomaktarihi.blogspot.com/2011/04/pomaklar-uzerine-dusunceler1.html. (Date of access: 16.11.2018)

78. Günsen, A. (2013). Pomaks as a Balkan community and evidence of Turkishness in their perceptions of identity. Journal of Balkan Research Institute, 2(1), 35.

81. http://pomaktarihi.blogspot.com/2007/04/kaypedilen-kimlikpomaklar.html.(Date of access: 16.11.2018)

83. Taşdelen, M., Şan K., Hira İ. (2008). On the customs of the gorillas: the first determinations, rock gora monument at the top of the hill, Editor: Ebubekir Sofuoğlu, Istanbul: Fsf Print Hause. 11–25.

84. Kalafat, Yaşar. (2006). The Turkish Folk Beliefs from the Balkans to Ulugh Turkestan, Berikan Publisher, Ankara.

86. http://pomaknews.com/?p=8057. (Date of access: 16.11.2018)

90. Çetin, N. (2011). Rumeli pomak muhacirlerinin kurduğu (iskân edildiği) osmaniye (kavakalan) köyü (izmir-bayındır-çınardibi) ve 1904 yılı osmanlı nüfus sayımı, http://fikiryolu.net. (Date of access: 14.11.2018)

92. Saygılı, H. (2014). Albanian Perception of the Ottomans and Turkey From the 20th Century to the Present. Wise Strategy, 6(10), 35–62.

93. Azimli, M. (2006). Albanian grand vizier husband (dervish) davut pasha, international albanian among the six centuries, Pristina Publisher, Kosovo.

94. Shehu, F. (2011). The influence of Islam on Albanian culture. Journal of Islam in Asia, 8, 389–408.

95. Zhelyazkova, A. (2000). Albanian ıdentities. Albania and the Albanian ıdentities. (Ed) antonina zhelyazkova. Sofia: International Center for Minority Studies. 9–63. 8, Eylül 2006, Priştina, Kosova.

96. Likaj, M. (2013). A study of the perception of social value of Albanian youth. Süleyman Demirel University Faculty of Arts and Sciences Journal of Social Sciences, 29.

97. http://www.nkfu.com/arnavutluk-dini-ve-dili-hakkinda-bilgi. (Date of access: 16.12.2018)

98. http://www.arnavut.com/mizac-ve-aile-yapisi/. (Date of access: 16.12.2018)

99. Doğan, A., & Garan, B. (2013). The memories are reflected in albania and albania. VIII. International Congress of the Grand Turkic Language, Albania Tirana, 427–451.

100. Koca, K. S. (2018). Common cultural elements seen in the transitional periods of the Turkish-macedonian-albanian-Bosnian communities in Macedonia. International Journal of Turkish Literature Culture Education, 7(2), 1085–1103.

102. Eker, S. (2006). On ethno-linguistic structure and Turkish language and culture in Bosnia. National Folklore, 72(18), 71–84.

103. Malcolm, N. (2002). Bosnia a Short History. London: Panbook.

104. İyiyol, F. (2010). Traces of the Turkish-Tekke Sufism in Bosnian Folk Culture. Unpublished PhD Thesis, Sakarya: Sakarya University, Institute of Social Sciences.

105. Nurkić, K. (2007). Islamization process in Bosnia and Herzegovina. Unpublished Master Thesis, Samsun: Ondokuz Mayis University, Institute of Social Sciences.

107. Tacoğlu, T. P., Arikan, G., & Sağir, A. (2012). Migration and cultural identity in Bosniak immigrants: the example of fevziye village. Electronic Turkish Studies, 7(1), 1941–1965.

108. Demir, G., & Bolat, S. (2017). Identity and belonging in Circassians. Journal of Sociological Studies/Sociology Conferences, (55), 1–42.

110. Aslan, C. (2005). Circassians in the Eastern Mediterranean, Adana: Caucasian Cultural Association Publications. 1–186.

111. Namitok, A. (2003). Çerkeslerin kökeni (Çev. A. Çeviker), Ankara: Kaf-Dav Yayınları.

112. Papşu, M. (2004 Mart), Anadolu'daki Abhazya, Atlas, Sayı: 132, 118–131.

115. Aslan, C., Sefer E. B., & M Papşu. (2011). Biz Çerkesler, Kafkas Dernekleri Federasyonu, Ankara, http://www.circassian.us/ Makaleler/Biz-Cerkesler.pdf.(Date of access 21.12.2018)

116. Yildiz, Y. (2018). Notes on the Circassian culture in the works of the 17th and 18th century Westerners. Abant İzzett Baysal

University Journal of the Institute of Social Sciences, 18(1, 18), 219–240.

117. Kalaycı, İ. (2015). Circassia (Circassians) in terms of history, culture and economics. Eurasian Studies, 47(1), 71–111.

118. Arayıcı, A. (2008). Stateless people of Europe: gypsies. First Edition. Istanbul: Kalkedon Publications.

119. Ünaldı, H. (2012). Living a cultural change in Turkey: gypsies. Batman University Journal of Life Science, 1(1), 615–626.

121. Kurtuluş, B. (2012). Gypsies as a Stateless People: Their Origins, Problems, Organizations, (Der.) Levent Ürer, Roman Olup Gypsy Stay, Istanbul: Melek Publications. 17–43.

122. Marsh, A. (2008). Ethnicity and identity: the origin of gypsies, (Jun.) Ebru Uzpeder, Savel Danova/Roussinova, Love Ozcelik, Sinan Gokcen, (trans.) Ezgi Taboğlu and Sezin Oney We are here!: Roma in Turkey, Discriminatory Practices and Rights Struggle, Istanbul: March Printing. 5–27.

126. Mezarcıoğlu, A. (2010). The Book of Gypsies. Istanbul: Cinius Publishing.

127. Kolukırık, S. (2009). Gypsies from past to present: cultural identity language history, istanbul: Ozan Yayıncılık. 59.

128. Yanıkdağ, T. (2012). Türkiye'de yaşayan romanların sorunları genel bir bakış, (Der.) Levent Ürer, Roman Olup Çingene Kalmak, İstanbul: Melek Yayınları. 247–270.

129. Aksu, M. (2003). Türkiye'de çingene olmak. 2. Baskı, İstanbul: Kesit Yayınları. 50.

131. Önder, Ö. (2009). Çingeneler. K. Emiroğlu, ve S. Aydın. içinde, Antropoloji Sözlüğü, Ankara: Bilim ve Sanat Yayınları. 196–201.

136. Özdemir, A. (2014). Working in Roma: poverty, sample of Sakarya Gazipaşa neighborhood, Master Thesis, Sakarya University, Social Sciences Institute, Sakarya.

137. Tanriverdi, G., Ünüvar, R., Yalçın, M., Acar, P., Yaman, B., Akçay, E., ... Sürer, M. (2012). Evaluate Gypsies' Living in Çanakkale According to "Purnell' Cultural Competence Model". Journal Of Anatolia Nursing And Health Sciences, 15(4). 243–253.

139. Campayo, J. G., & Alda, M. (2007). Illness behaviors and cultural characteristics of the gypsy population in Spain. Actas Espanolas Psiquiatria, 35(1), 59–66.

141. Genç, Y., Taylan, H. H., & Barış, İ. (2015). The role of social exclusion in the educational process and academic achievement of Roma children. The Journal of Academic Social Science Studies, 33, 79–97.

142. Gökçen, S., & ve Öney, S. (2008). In Turkey, Roma and Nationalism (Jun.) Ebru Uzpeder, Savel Danova/Roussinova, Love Ozcelik, Sinan Gokcen, (trans.) Ezgi Taboğlu and Sezin Oney, We are Here!: Roma in Turkey, Discriminatory Practices and Rights Struggle, Istanbul: March Printing. 129–135.

143. Ceyhan, S. (2003). A case study of Gypsy/Roma identity construction in Edirne. Unpublished Master's Thesis. Ankara: Middle East Technical University, Institute of Social Sciences. 147–54.

146. Özkan, A. R. (2006). Marriage among the Gypsies of Turkey. The Social Science Journal, 43(3), 461–70.

148. Cleemput, P. V., & Parry, G. Health status of Gypsy travellers. Journal of Public Health Medicine, 23(2), 129–34.

150. Molnár, Á., Ádám, B., Antova, T., Bosak, L., Dimitrov, P., Mileva, H., ... & Kósa, K. (2012). Health impact assessment of Roma housing policies in Central and Eastern Europe: A comparative analysis. Environmental Impact Assessment Review, 33(1), 7–14.

151. Kabakchieva, E., Amirkhanian, Y. A., Kelly, J. A., McAuliffe, T. L., & Vassileva, S. (2002). High levels of sexual HIV/STD risk behaviors among Roma (Gypsy) men in Bulgaria: pattern and predictors of risk in a representative community sample. International Journal of STD & AIDS, 13(3), 184–91.

152. Kelly, J. A., Amirkhanian, Y. A., Kabakchieva, E., Csepe, P., Seal, D. W., Antonova, R., Mihayiov, A., & Gyukits, G. (2004). Gender roles and HIV sexual risk vulnerability of Roma (gypsies) men and woman in Bulgaria and Hungary; an ethnographic study. AIDS Care, 16(2), 231–245.

153. Sutherland, A. (1992). Cross-cultural medicine. A decade later. Gypsies and health care. West J Med, 157(3), 276–280.

154. Campayo, J. G. (2007). Alda M. Illness behaviors and cultural characteristics of the gypsy population in Spain. Actas Espanolas Psiquiatria, 35(1), 59–66.

158. Özyazıcıoğlu, N., & Öncel, S. (2011). Cultural approaches in child care. Intercultural Nursing. First Edition. Istanbul: İstanbul Medical. 203–239.

160. Cleemput, P. V., Parry, G. (2001). Health status of Gypsy travellers. Journal of Public Health Medicine, 23(2), 129–134.

161. Berberoğlu, U., Eskiocak, M., Ekukulu, G., & Saltık, A. (2001). The use of novels and others in primary health care center in Edirne province. Society and Physician, 16(6), 470–475.

163. Yazıcı, M. (2011). The Understanding of Alevism: Sociological Analysis of the Alevi Sayings and Gülbangs in Kavalcık. Unpublished PhD Thesis. Firat University, Institute of Social Sciences, Elazığ/Turkey.

164. Dalkıran, S. (2002). An experiment on the Alevi identity and the Anatolian flame. EKEV Academy of Journal, 6(10), 95–118.

165. Üçer, C. (2005a). Worship life in traditional Alevism and the approaches of the Alevi to basic Islamic prayer. Journal of Neuroscience Academic Research, 5(3), 161–189.

166. Gümüş, N. (2011). Women in Alevism: The perception of the women of the women in the Şahkulu Sultan Dervish. Unpublished Master's Thesis. Dumlupınar University, Institute of Social Sciences, Kütahya.

167. Özcan, A. K. (2013). A field study on the Muslims of Alevis. Tunceli University Journal of Social Sciences, 2(3), 27–44.

168. Taşğın, A. (2009). Cem, Cemevi and Functions. Alevi-Bektashi Culture from Past to Present. (Ed) Ahmet Yasar January. Ankara: Ministry of Culture and Tourism Publications. 211–225.

170. Şahin, B. (2015). Alevi Identity and Revolt Teaching. Journal of International Social Research, 8(39), 539–548.

171. Salman, C. (2017). Turkey location of the flame experience in migration and urbanization: a periodization proposal. Journal of Faculty of Economics and Administrative Sciences, (2017/ Special Issue), 24–51.

173. Gezik, E. (2013). Alevi Kurds: religious, ethnic and political issues. istanbul: Communication Publications. 1–27.

174. Aktaş, A. (1999a). Changes in the family structure in the transformation process of the rural. Turkish Culture and Journal of Hacı Bektaş Velî Research, 12, 1–60.

176. http://hasanharmanci.blogcu.com/hizir-alevi-ekonomi-politigi/20418896 (Date of access: 15.06.2018).

177. Yeşilyurt, T. (2003). Faith dimension of Alevi-Bektashism. Islamiyat VI, 3, 13–30.

178. Bulut, H. İ., & ve Çetin, M. (2011). Religious Beliefs and Experiences Of. e-Makalat Journal of Sectional Research, 3(2), 165.

180. Üçer, C. (2005b). Traditional Alevism in Tokat. Ankara: Ankara School Publications.

181. Şahin, M. (2011). Concept of community and family in Alevi tradition. Journal of Kalam Research, 9(1), 263–284.

182. Aktaş, A. (1999b). The sociological evaluation of the incidence of flames in urban environment and the frequency of applying belief rituals. Ankara: Gazi University Turkish Culture and Hacı Bektaş Parent Research Center Publication. 449–482.

183. Çınar, F., & ve Eti Aslan, F. (2018). Evaluation of Anatolian Alevi people living in Istanbul with "Purnell' Cultural Competence Model". Journal of Human Sciences, 15(1), 98–111.

184. Keskin, M. (2003). The beliefs and rituals related to death in the flames of the Sarısaltık quarry (Tunceli Karacaköy Example). Erciyes University Journal of Social Sciences Institute, 1(15), 115–130.

191. Yalçın, H. (2016). Child rearing and position of women in Alevi culture. Turkish Culture and Journal of Hacı Bektaş Veli Research, 79, 79–94.

192. Rençber, Fevzi. (2012). The historical origin of the "Cem House" in the Alevi tradition. Journal of Religious Studies, 12(3), 73–86.

193. Albayrak, A., & ve Çapcıoğlu, İ. (2006). Folk beliefs and practices in a middle anadolu village in the Ahl-i Sunnah tradition. Religious Studies, 8(24), 107–132.

194. Bahadır, İ. (2005). Women dervishes in Alevi and Sunni dervishes. Istanbul: Water Publishing House.

195. Dierl, A. J. (1991). Anatolian Alevism. Fahrettin Yiğit (trans.) Istanbul: Ant Publications. 157.

196. Menemencioğlu, B. (2011). Women in Bektashi and Alevi Culture. Turkish Culture and Journal of Hacı Bektaş Velî Research, 60, 129–140.

197. Ünlüsoy, K. (2009). An Investigation on Women in the Alevi-Bektashi Tradition., II/2, 55–90.

198. Kaya, H. (1995). The rules of Alevism. Istanbul: Engin Publishing. 39–45.

199. Kaplan, A. (2003). Family and kinship institution in Aleppo, Alevism. Istanbul: Book Publishing.

200. Noyan, B. (1995). Bektashism What is Alevism? (3rd Edition). Istanbul: Ant/Can Publishing.

203. Süleymanov, A. (2009). Family and marital relationships in contemporary Turkish societies. Journal of Social Policy Studies, 5(17), 7-17.

204. http://www.alevicanlar.net/konu/alevilikte-aile-kavrami.8039/ (Date of access: 17.06.2018).

205. Gül, İ. (2014). Alevism as a social system. Hünkâr Alevîlik Bektashism Academic Research Journal, 1(1), 67.

206. Korkmaz, E. (2008). Anatolian Alevism, Philosophy-Faith-Doctrine-Erkanı. Istanbul: Berfin Publications.

207. Çamuroğlu, R. (2010). Alevi revival in Turkey, contrasts. The Alevi Identity (3rd Edition), Olsson T., Özdalga E., Raudvere C. (ed.), Bilge Kurt Torun, Hayati Torun (trans.), Istanbul: History Foundation Yurt Publications.

208. Gümüş, N. (2011) Women in Alevism: Perception of Alevi Women in Şahkulu Sultan Dergâhı. Unpublished Master's Thesis. Dumlupınar University, Institute of Social Sciences, Kütahya.

209. Özcan, H. (2005). The value of human beings in the culture of Alevi Bektashi influencing Asian societies. I.International Symposium of Asian Philosophical Society, Istanbul.

210. Ulusoy, Y. D., Karşıcı, G., ve Selçuk, A. (2013). In The Faith System Of The Beydili Village Of Sivas. Journal of Human Sciences, 2(2), 22–43.

213. Demirbilek, M. (2007). Children in Alevi Culture. Journal of Society and Social Work, 18(2), 65–75.

214. TÜİK- Turkey Statistical Institute. (2014). Child with statistics. Ankara: Turkey Statistics Institution Press. 72.

215. Güleç, C. (2000). Transcultural view of health concepts in Anatolian culture. Journal of Clinical Psychiatry, 3(1), 34–39.

217. Ergun, P. (2011). Alevism on the mythological origins of rabbit belief in Bektashism. Turkish Culture and Journal of Hacı Bektaş Veli Research, 60, 281–306.

221. Kılıç, S., Altuncu, A., & Gaspak, A. (2016). Beliefs and practices related to birth in flames living in Anatolian countryside (Haçova Case). Electronic Turkish Studies, 11(17), 431–446.

222. Büyükokutan, A. (2005). Muğla region A research on folk literature and folklore products of Alevi Turkmens. Master Thesis. Balıkesir University Institute of Social Sciences Department of Turkish Language and Literature. 327–417

223. Yıldırım, E. (2010). A sociological study on the beliefs and practices of the transition period in the Tunceli region. EKEV Academy Journal, 14(42), 17–32.

224. Selçuk, A. (2004). A phenomenological approach to the beliefs and practices of planners about birth. Turkology Researches, 16(16), 163–178.

228. Yazlak, Y. (2011). Haçova village culture and history. Malatya Haçova Village Culture and Solidarity Association, 1, 3–5.

234. Örnek, S. V. (2000). Turkish Folklore, Ankara: Ministry of Culture Publications. 162–163.

235. Karaağaç, G., & ve Alacain, Ş. (2004). Our house in Ortaca. Muğla: Anıl Ofset-Tipo Typography. 362.

236. Şöhret, D. Ü. (2004). Folk medicine in Fethiye and the beliefs about it, Book of Muğla. Prepared by: Ali Abbas Cinar, Izmir: Printer Offset Printing. 297.

241. Purnell, L. (2008). Transcultural diversity and health care. In: Purnell L, Paulkanca BJ, eds. Transcultural health care: A culturally competent approach. 3rd ed. Philadelphia: F.A. Davis Company. 19–55.

243. Turkish Statistical Institute TÜİK. (2017). Employment and Household data. http://www.tuik.gov.tr/PreTablo.do?alt_id=1007. (Date of access: 17.12.2018)

About the Author

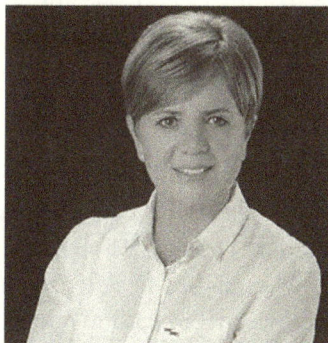

Dr. Fatma Eti Aslan
Dean of Faculty of Health Sciences at Bahcesehir Universityi, Istanbul, Turkey Professor Eti Aslan obtained her nursing license from the Istanbul University Florence Nightingale Nursing School in 1986, her master degree from Istanbul University Institute of Health Sciences Department of Nursing in 1988, her doctoral degree from Istanbul University Institute of Health Sciences Department of Medical Surgical Nursing in 1992. She worked at Cerrahpasa Hospital as a nurse for three years and then at Marmara University as an assistant professor between 1993–1999, as an associate professor between 1999–2006 and as a professor between 2006–2009. She is still working at Bahcesehir University Faculty of Health Sciences as a head of Nursing program and as a dean of faculty. Professor Eti Aslan managed 43 master's thesis and four (4) doctorate thesis until now. She is an author of four (4) nursing books, editor of 12 books, author of lots of chapters and she also has 34 international SCI, SSCI scientific papers, 98 national papers and 53 international congress participation. She continues to teach continuously.

Dr. Fadime Çınar
Fadime ÇINAR graduated from Istanbul University, Department of Nursing in 1999. During her master's and doctoral studies, she worked as a senior executive in education and research up to twenty two years. Her areas of expertise are surgical nursing, operating room nursing and

research methods. Her master degree from Marmara University Institute of Health Sciences Department of Nursing in 2007, her doctoral degree from Bahçeşehir University Institute of Health Sciences Department of Nursing in 2019. Dr. Çınar has many international publications in the field of nursing and health management.

* * * *

This book was created in the light of these experiences considering how individuals in different cultures in Turkey evaluate the concepts of health and disease. It is important to know the cultural characteristics of the community to allow individuals and societies to participate by accepting this service in order to provide them with the desired level of health care. The conditions that are culturally important are generally overlooked in the presentation of health services. Providing a proper cultural health care, understanding the dimensions of culture, leading to a holistic approach more than biophysicality, increasing knowledge, changing approaches and improving clinical skills. This book is written by people who have experienced it in order to guide their health service servers. I believe that all readers will bring a scientific view of the pain and thank everyone who contributed to it.